Simple Anti Inflammatory Recipe Collections

Affordable and Delicious Meat

Recipes to Boost Your Metabolism

Zac Gibson

Table of Contents

Herby Chicken Fillets

Prep Time:
15 minutes
Serve: 6

Ingredients:

- 1 1/2 pounds chicken fillets
- 1 1/2 tablespoons olive oil
- 1/2 teaspoon ground black pepper
- 1 teaspoon kosher salt
- 1 stick butter
- 2 teaspoons apple cider vinegar
- 1/3 cup chopped fresh cilantro
- 2 tablespoons finely minced shallots
- 1 teaspoon finely minced garlic

Directions:

1.Preheat a skillet over moderate heat. Add the olive oil. Fry the chicken fillets for around 10 minutes until they are brown.

2.In a bowl mix together the salt, pepper, butter, apple cider vinegar, cilantro, shallots and garlic.

3.Serve the chicken fillets with the herby sauce.

Nutrition: Calories 258.6, Protein 15.2g, Fat 20.2g Carbs 4g Sugar 1.5g

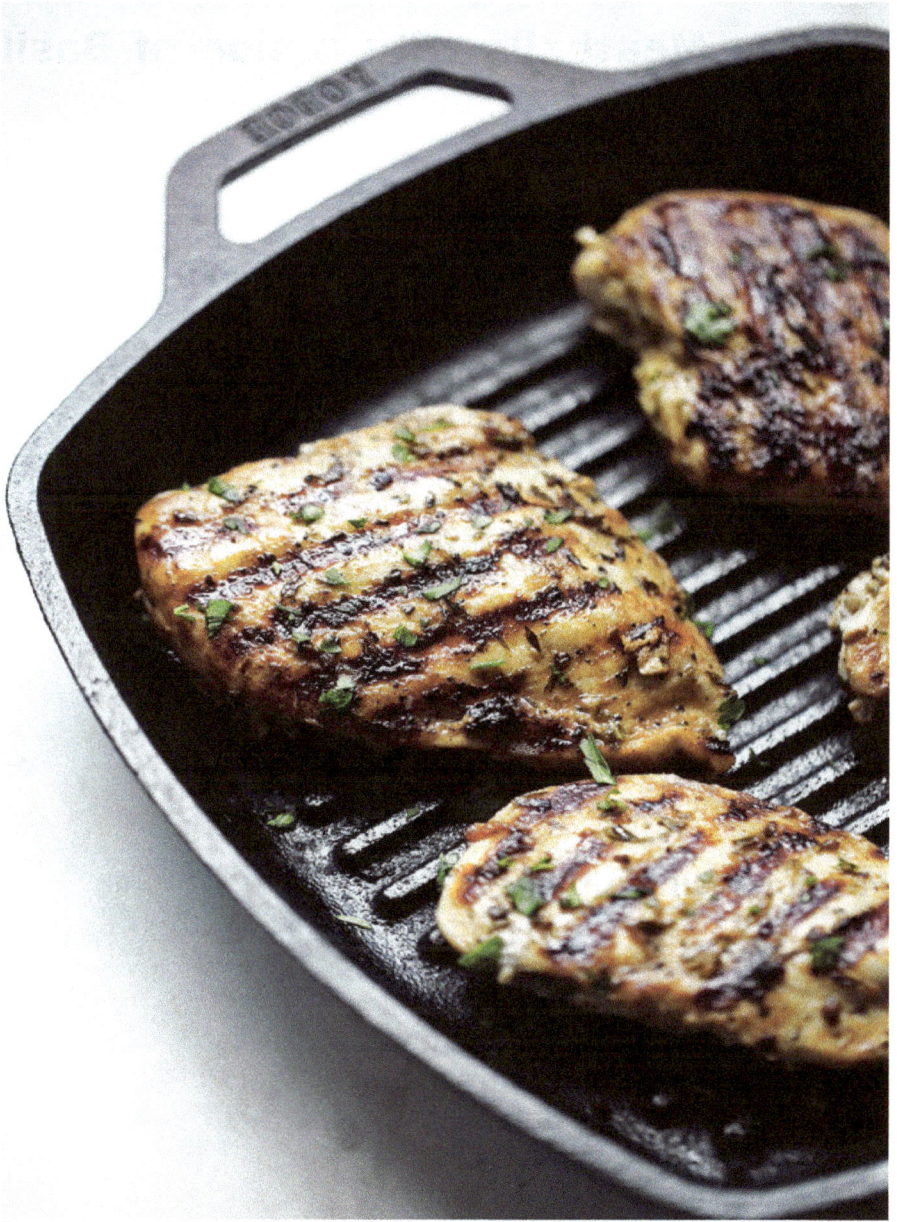

Turkey Meatballs with a side of Basil Chutney

Prep Time:
30 minutes
Serve: 6

Ingredients:

- 2 tablespoons olive oil
- 1 1/2 pounds ground turkey
- 1/4 teaspoon ground black pepper
- 1/2 teaspoon sea salt
- ½ teaspoon celery seeds
- 1/4 teaspoon dried thyme
- 1/2 teaspoon onion powder
- 1/2 teaspoon garlic powder
- 3 tablespoons flax seed meal
- 1/2 teaspoons paprika
- ½ cup grated Parmesan cheese
- 2 small-sized eggs, lightly beaten

For the Basil Chutney:

- 1/2 cup fresh basil leaves
- 1/2 cup coriander leaves
- 2 tablespoons fresh lemon juice
- 1 teaspoon grated fresh ginger root
- 2 tablespoons water
- 2 tablespoons olive oil
- Salt and pepper, to taste
- 1 tablespoon minced green chili

Directions:

1.Mix all the meatball ingredients. Form into 16 balls and put to one side.

2.Preheat a skillet over medium heat and then heat the olive oil.

3.Fry the meatballs for 7 -8 minutes, making sure that all sides are browned.

4.Then make the chutney. Put the basil leaves, coriander leaves, lemon juice, ginger, olive oil, salt, pepper and chili into a food processor and blend.

Nutrition: Calories 260, Protein 25.4g, Fat 15g, Carbs 6g, Sugar 2.1g

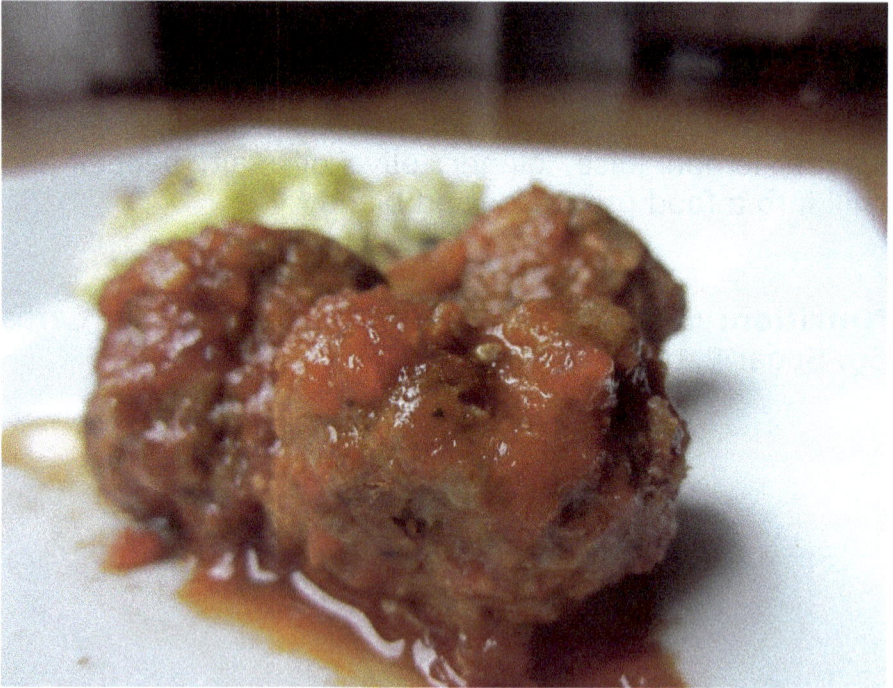

Asian Saucy Chicken

Prep Time:
25 minutes
Serve: 4

Ingredients:

- 1 tablespoon sesame oil
- 4 chicken legs
- 1/4 cup Shaoxing wine
- 2 tablespoons brown erythritol
- 1/4 cup spicy tomato sauce

Directions:

1.Heat the sesame oil in a wok over medium-high heat. Fry the chicken until golden in color; reserve.

2.Add Shaoxing wine to deglaze the pan.

3.Add in erythritol and spicy tomato sauce, and bring the mixture to a boil.

4.Then, immediately reduce the heat to medium-low.

5.Let it simmer for about 10 minutes until the sauce coats the back of a spoon.

6.Add the chicken back to the wok.

7.Continue to cook until the chicken is sticky and golden or about 4 minutes.

Nutrition: 367 Calories; 14.7g Fat; 3.5g Carbs; 51.2g Protein; 1.1g Fiber

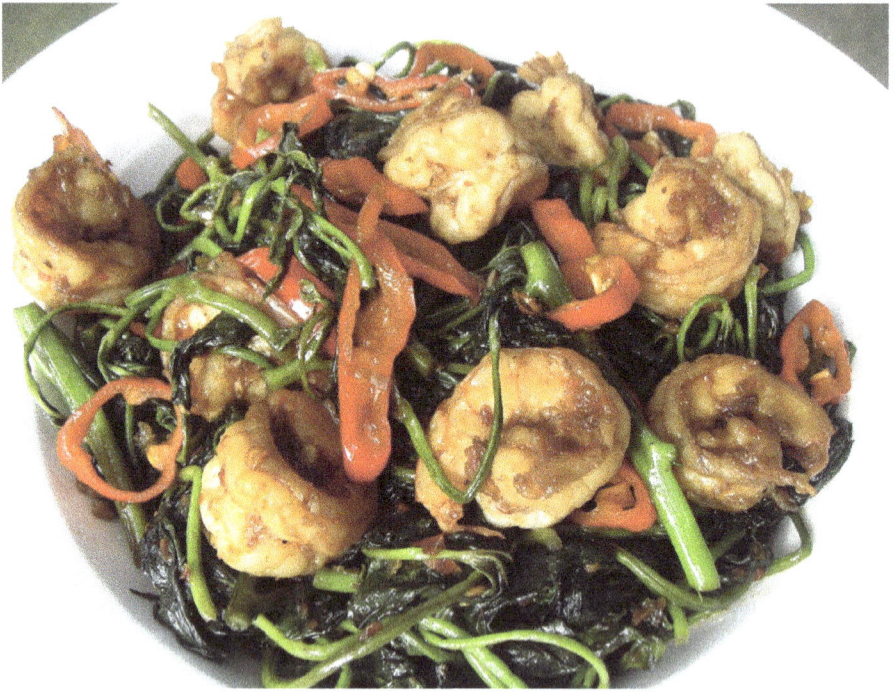

Duck Stew Olla Tapada

Prep Time:
30 minutes
Serve: 3

Ingredients:

- 1 red bell pepper, deveined and chopped
- 1 pound duck breasts, boneless, skinless, and chopped into small chunks
- 1/2 cup chayote, peeled and cubed
- 1 shallot, chopped
- 1 teaspoon Mexican spice mix

Directions:

1.In a clay pot, heat 2 teaspoons of canola oil over a medium-high flame. Sauté the peppers and shallot until softened about 4 minutes.

2.Add in the remaining ingredients; pour in 1 ½ cups of water or chicken bone broth.

3.Once your mixture starts boiling, reduce the heat to medium-low.

4.Let it simmer, partially covered, for 18 to 22 minutes, until cooked through.

Nutrition: 228 Calories; 9.5g Fat; 3.3g Carbs; 30.6g Protein; 1g Fiber

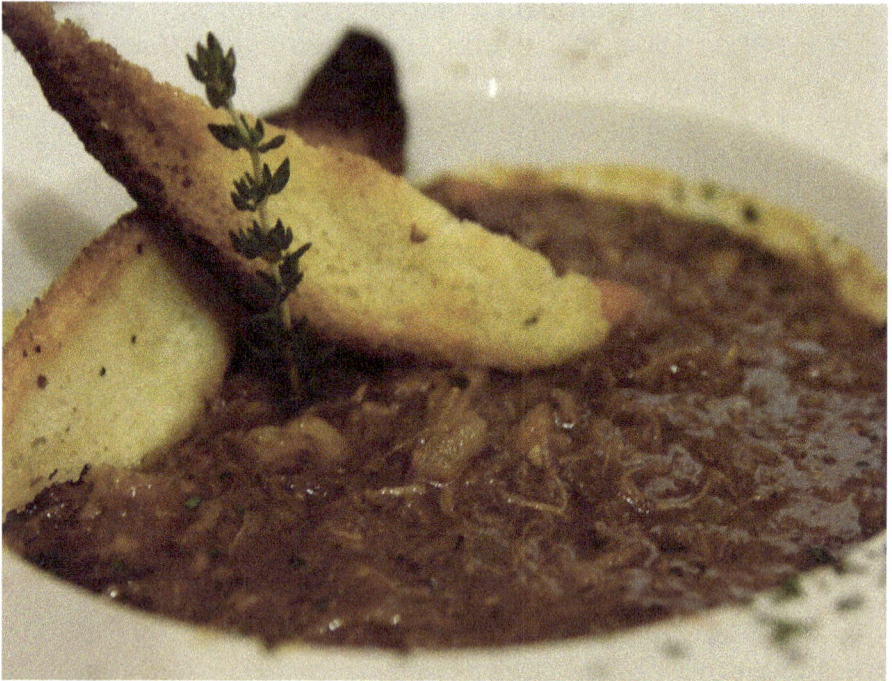

Cheesy Ranch Chicken

Prep Time:
20 minutes
Serve: 4

Ingredients:

- 2 chicken breasts
- 1/2 tablespoon ranch seasoning mix
- 4 slices bacon, chopped
- 1/2 cup Monterey-Jack cheese, grated
- 4 ounces Ricotta cheese, room temperature

Directions:

1.Preheat your oven to 360 degrees F.

2.Rub the chicken with ranch seasoning mix.

3.Heat a saucepan over medium-high flame. Now, sear the chicken for about 8 minutes.

4.Lower the chicken into a lightly greased casserole dish.

5.Top with cheese and bacon and bake in the preheated oven for about 10 minutes until hot and bubbly. Serve with freshly snipped scallions, if desired.

Nutrition: 295 Calories; 19.5g Fat; 2.9g Carbs; 25.5g Protein; 0.4g Fiber

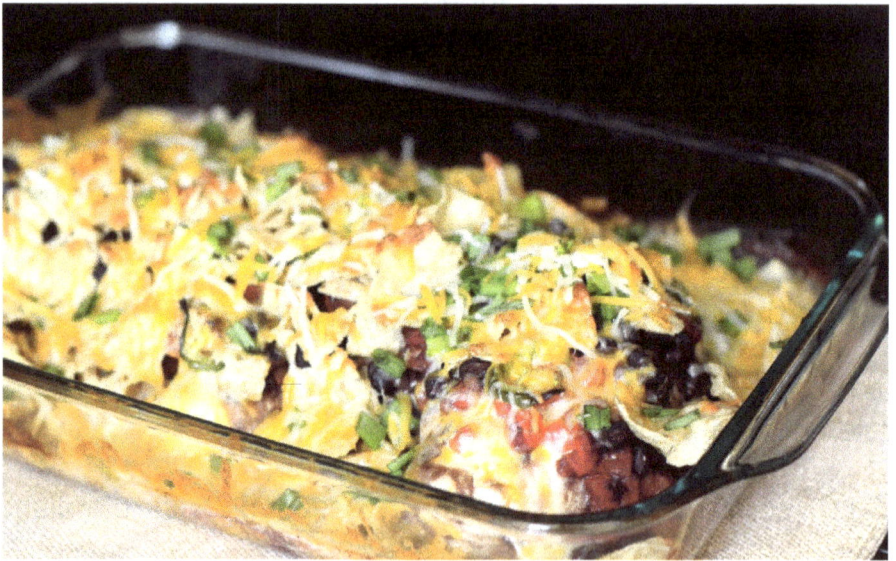

Turkey Crust Meatza

Prep Time:
35 minutes
Serve: 4

Ingredients:

- ½ pound ground turkey
- 2 slices Canadian bacon
- 1 tomato, chopped
- 1 tablespoon pizza spice mix
- 1 cup Mozzarella cheese, grated

Directions:

1.Mix the ground turkey and cheese; season with salt and black pepper and mix until everything is well combined.

2.Press the mixture into a foil-lined baking pan. Bake in the preheated oven at 380 degrees F for 25 minutes.

3.Top the crust with Canadian bacon, tomato, and pizza spice mix. Continue to bake for a further 8 minutes.

4.Let it rest a couple of minutes before slicing and.

Nutrition: 360 Calories; 22.7g Fat; 5.9g Carbs; 32.6g Protein; 0.7g Fiber

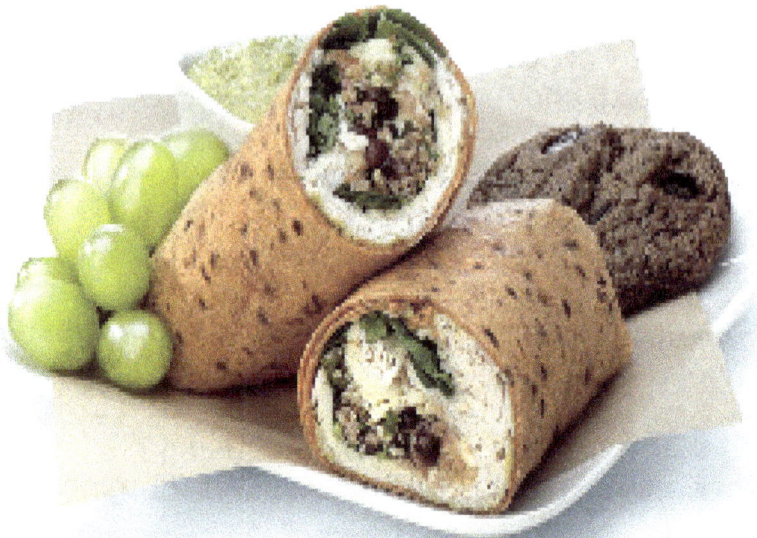

Simple Turkey Goulash

Prep Time:
45 minutes
Serve: 6

Ingredients:

- 2 tablespoons olive oil
- 1 large-sized leek, chopped
- 2 cloves garlic, minced
- 2 pounds turkey thighs, skinless, boneless and chopped
- 2 celery stalks, chopped

Directions:

1.In a clay pot, heat 2 olive oil over a medium-high flame. Then, cook the leeks until tender and translucent.

2.Then, continue to sauté the garlic for 30 seconds to 1 minute.

3.Stir in the turkey, celery, and 4 cups of water. Once your mixture starts boiling, let it simmer, partially covered, for about 40 minutes.

Nutrition: 220 Calories; 7.4g Fat; 2.7g Carbs; 35.5g Protein; 1g Fiber

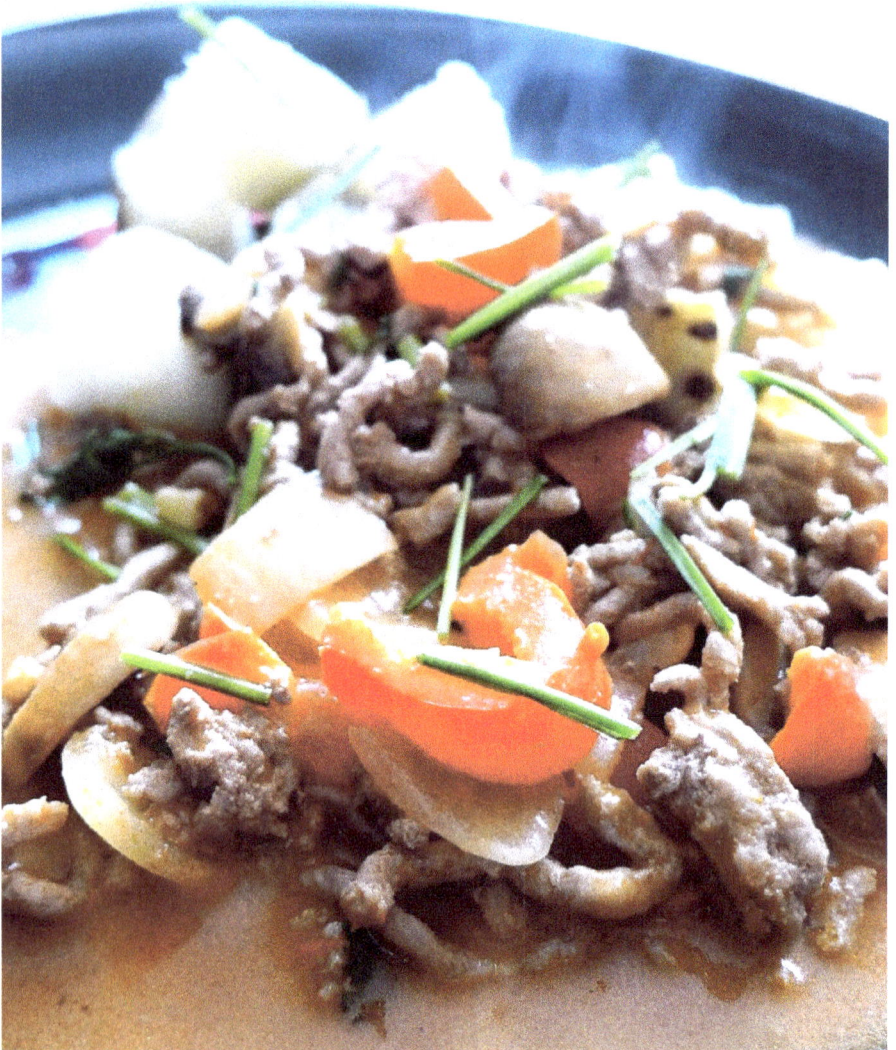

Fajita with Zucchini

Prep Time:
20 minutes
Serve: 4

Ingredients:

- 1 red onion, sliced
- 1 teaspoon Fajita seasoning mix
- 1 pound turkey cutlets
- 1 zucchini, spiralized
- 1 chili pepper, chopped

Directions:

1.In a nonstick skillet, heat 1 tablespoon of the olive oil over a medium-high flame.

2.Cook the turkey cutlets for 6 to 7 minutes on each side. Slice the meat into strips and reserve.

3.Heat another tablespoon of olive oil and sauté the onion and chili pepper until they are just tender. Sprinkle with Fajita seasoning mix.

4.Add in the zucchini and the reserved turkey; let it cook for 4 minutes more or until everything is cooked through. Serve with 1/2 cup of salsa, if desired. Enjoy!

Nutrition: 212 Calories; 9.2g Fat; 5.6g Carbs; 26g Protein; 1.2g Fiber

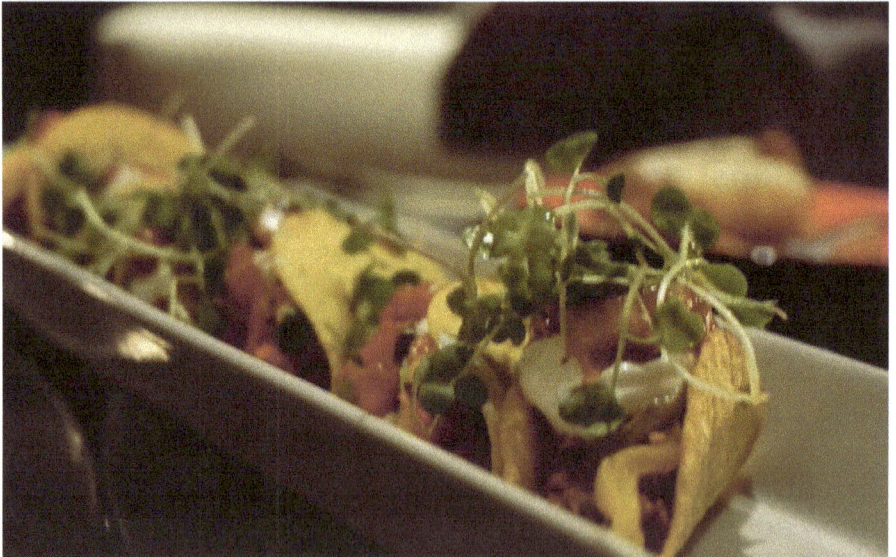

Easiest Turkey Meatballs Ever

Prep Time:
1 hour 20 minutes
Serve: 4

Ingredients:

- 1 egg, whisked
- 4 spring onions, finely chopped
- 1/2 cup parmesan cheese, grated
- 1 tablespoon Italian spice mix
- 1 pound ground turkey

Directions:

1.Thoroughly combine all ingredients. Roll the turkey mixture into balls and place them in your refrigerator for 1 hour.

2.In a cast-iron skillet, heat 2 tablespoons of olive oil over medium-high heat.

3.Sear the meatballs for 12 minutes or until nicely browned on all sides.

Nutrition: 366 Calories; 27.7g Fat; 3g Carbs; 25.9g Protein; 0.5g Fiber

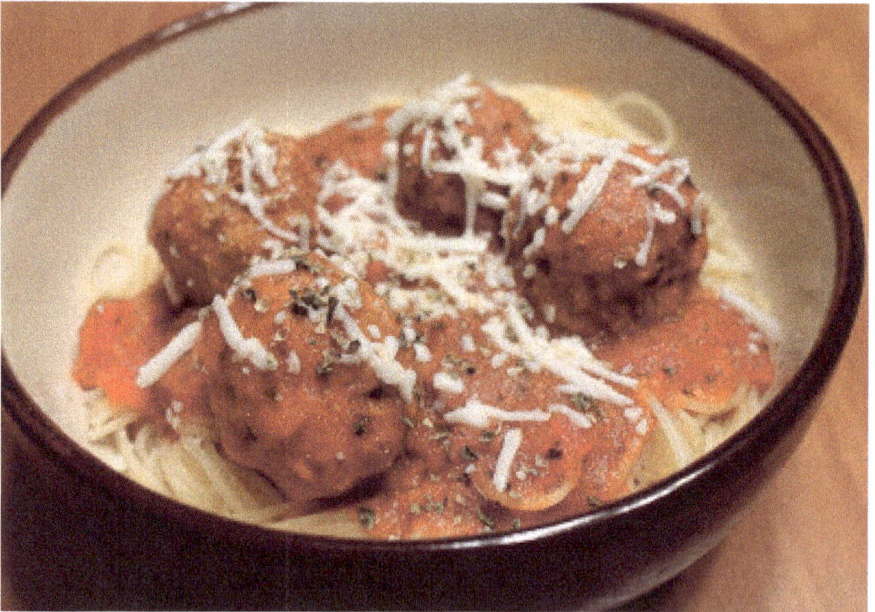

Greek-Style Chicken Drumettes

Prep Time:
30 minutes
Serve: 2

Ingredients:

- 1 tablespoon olive oil
- 6 Kalamata olives, pitted and sliced
- 1 pound chicken drumettes
- 6 ounces tomato sauce
- 1 teaspoon Greek seasoning blend

Directions:

1.Rub the chicken drumettes with Greek seasoning blend.

2.In a nonstick skillet, heat the olive oil over medium-high flame. Sear the chicken for about 10 minutes until nicely brown.

3.Add in the olives and tomato sauce. Stir and continue to cook, partially covered, for about 18 minutes until everything is thoroughly heated. Bon appétit!

Nutrition: 341 Calories; 14.3g Fat; 3.6g Carbs; 47g Protein; 1.1g Fiber

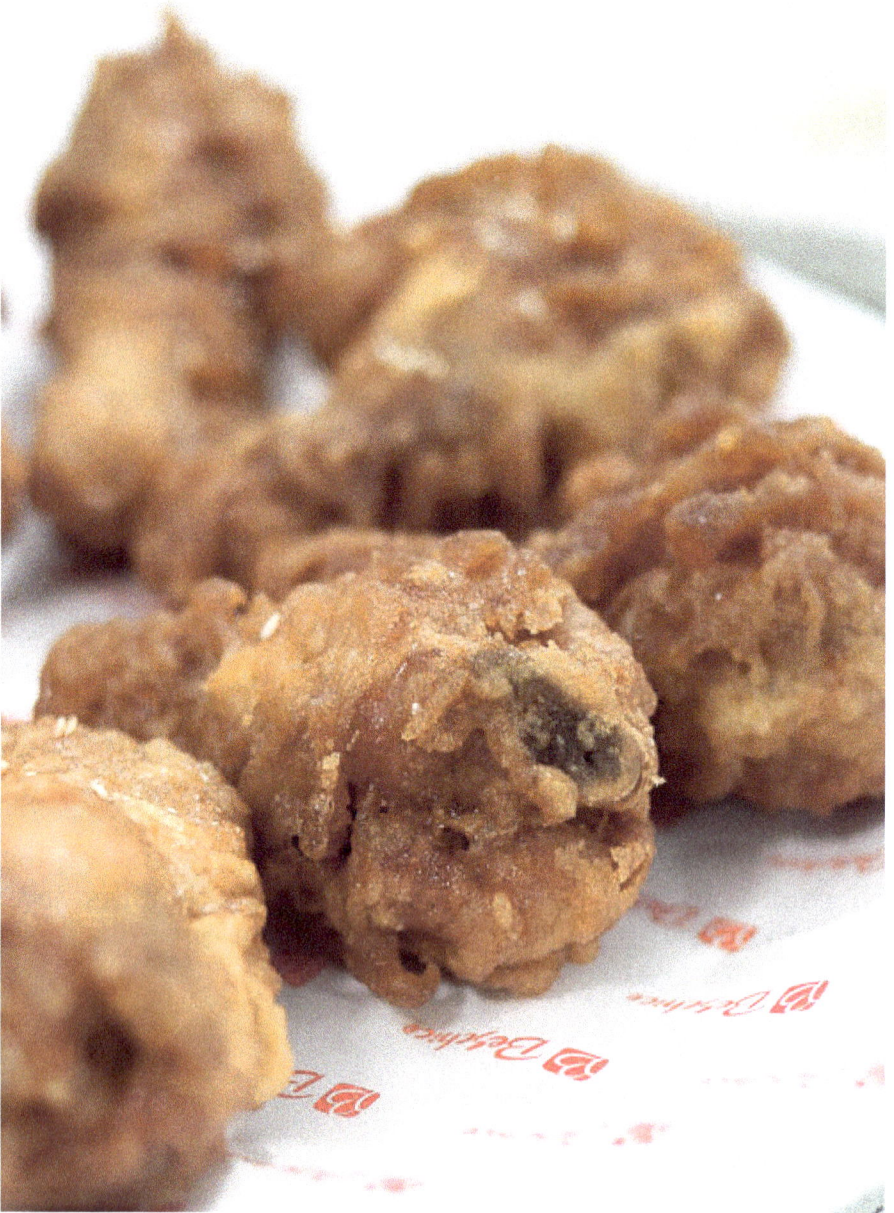

Chicken Tawook Salad

Prep Time:
20 minutes
Serve: 2

Ingredients:

- 2 chicken breasts
- 4 tablespoons apple cider vinegar
- 1 cup grape tomatoes, halved
- 1 Lebanese cucumber, thinly sliced
- 2 tablespoons extra-virgin olive oil

Directions:

1.Preheat a grill to medium-high and oil a grill grate. Grill the chicken for about 13 minutes, turing them over a few times.

2.Slice the chicken into the bite-sized chunks and transfer them to a bowl.

3.Add in the vinegar, tomatoes, cucumber, and olive oil. Toss to combine well.

Nutrition: 403 Calories; 18g Fat; 5.3g Carbs; 51.6g Protein; 1.6g Fiber

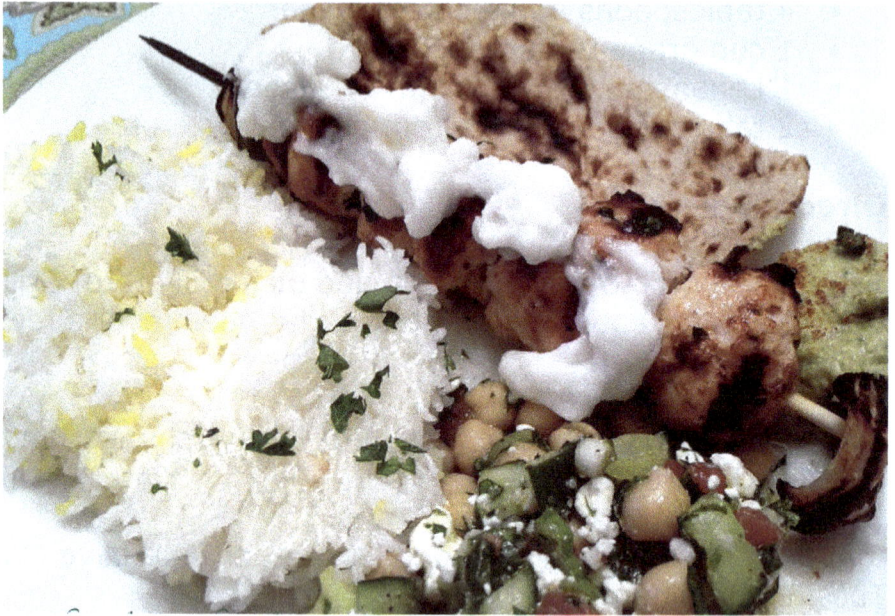

Greek Chicken with Peppers

Prep Time:
20 minutes
Serve: 2

Ingredients:

- 2 chicken drumsticks, boneless and skinless
- 2 bell peppers, deveined and halved
- 1 small chili pepper, finely chopped
- 2 tablespoons Greek aioli
- 6 Kalamata olives, pitted

Directions

1.Rub the chicken with 1 tablespoon of extra-virgin olive oil. Season with salt and black pepper to taste.

2.Grill the chicken drumsticks for 8 to 9 minutes; add the bell peppers and grill them for a further 6 minutes.

3.Place the meat and peppers in a bowl; add in chili pepper and Greek aioli.

4.Top with Kalamata olives and serve.

Nutrition: 403 Calories; 31.4g Fat; 5g Carbs; 24.5g Protein; 1.1g Fiber

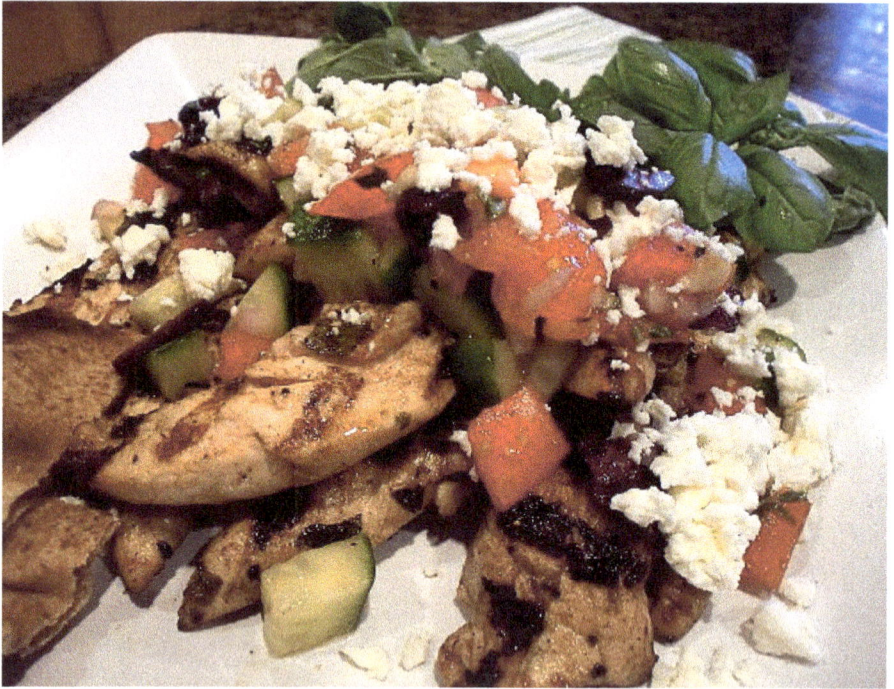

Colorful Chicken Chowder

Prep Time:
50 minutes
Serve: 6

Ingredients:

- 1 tablespoon olive oil
- 6 chicken wings
- 1 cup mixed frozen vegetables (celery, onions, and pepper
- 1 tablespoon poultry seasoning mix
- 1 whole egg

Directions:

1.Heat the olive oil in a heavy-bottomed pot over medium-high heat.

2.Then, brown the chicken for 10 minutes or until no longer pink; set them aside.

3.Then, cook the vegetables in the pan drippings until they are crisp-tender.

4.Season with poultry seasoning mix and turn the heat to medium-low; continue to simmer for a further 40 minutes or until everything is thoroughly cooked.

5.Chop the chicken and discard the fat and bones.

6.Whisk the egg into the cooking liquid. Add the reserved chicken back to the pot. Taste and adjust the seasonings.

Nutrition: 283 Calories; 18.9g Fat; 2.6g Carbs; 25.4g Protein; 0.5g Fiber

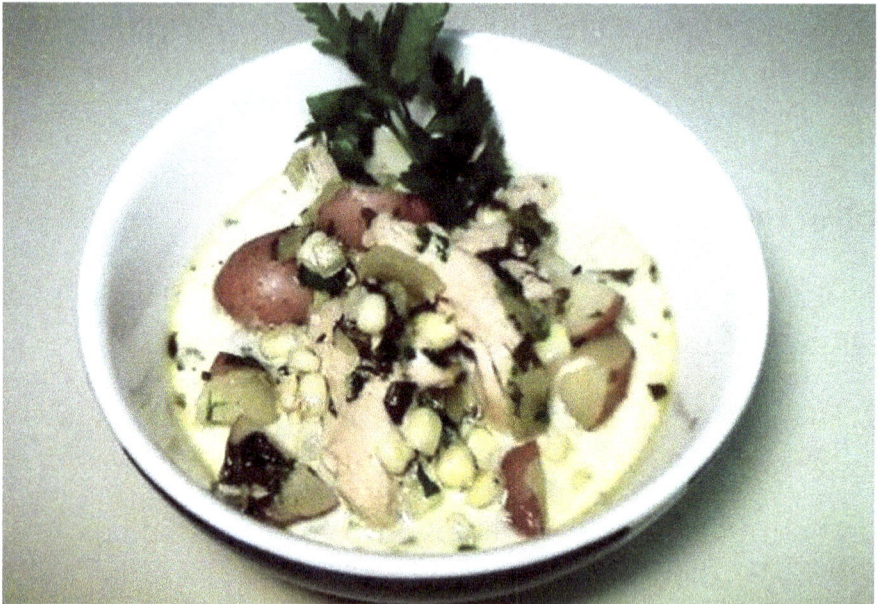

Chicken Frittata with Asiago Cheese and Herbs

Prep Time:
30 minutes
Serve: 4

Ingredients:

- 1 pound chicken breasts, cut into small strips
- 4 slices of bacon
- 1 cup Asiago cheese, shredded
- 6 eggs
- 1/2 cup yogurt

Directions

1.Preheat an oven-proof skillet. Then, fry the bacon until crisp and reserve.

2.Then, cook the chicken for about 8 minutes or until no longer pink in the pan drippings.

3.Add the reserved bacon back to the skillet.

4.In a mixing dish, thoroughly combine the eggs and yogurt; season with Italian spice mix.

5.Pour the egg mixture over the chicken and bacon. Top with cheese and bake in the preheated oven at 380 degrees F for 22 minutes until hot and bubbly.

6.Let it rest a couple of minutes before slicing.

Nutrition: 484 Calories; 31.8g Fat; 5.8g Carbs; 41.9g Protein; 0.7g Fiber

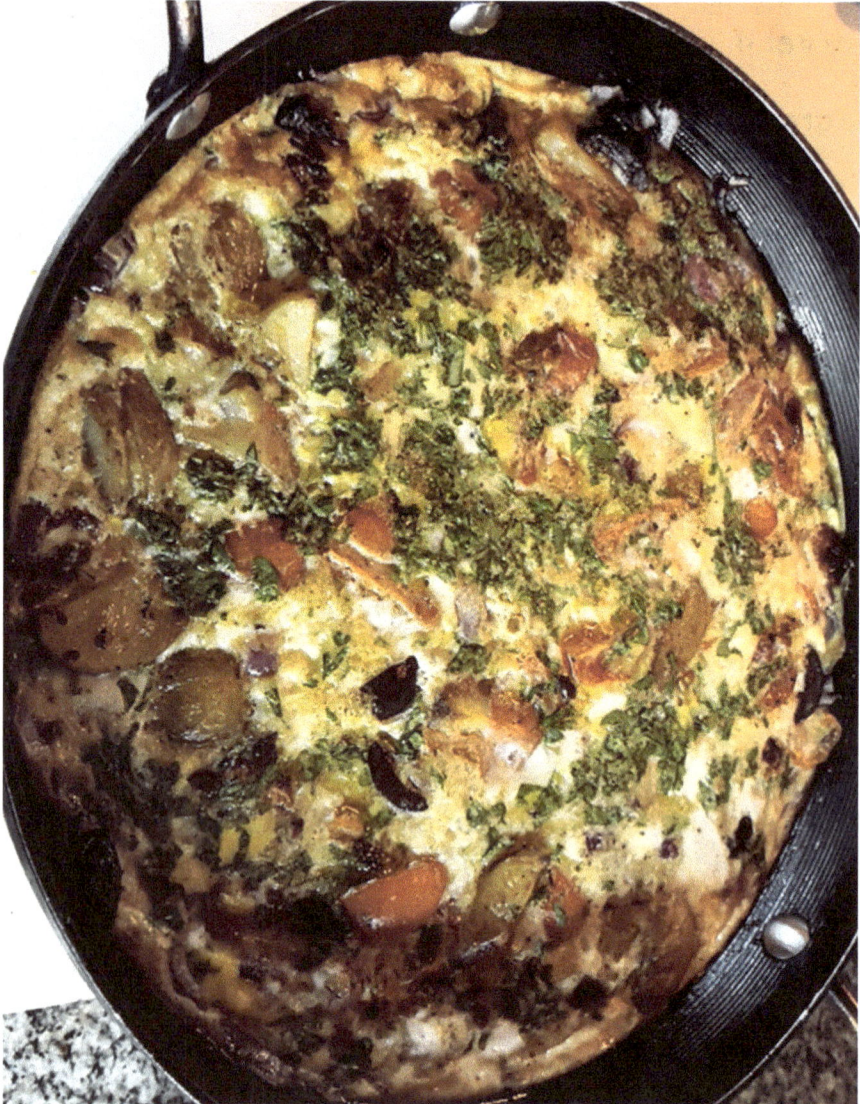

Stuffed Chicken with Sauerkraut and Cheese

Prep Time:
35 minutes
 Serve: 5

Ingredients:

- 5 chicken cutlets
- 1 cup Romano cheese, shredded
- 2 garlic cloves, minced
- 5 Italian peppers, deveined and chopped
- 5 tablespoons sauerkraut

Directions:

1.Spritz a baking pan with 1 tablespoon of the olive oil.

2.Brush the chicken with another tablespoon of olive oil.

3.Season the chicken with Italian spice mix. You can spread Dijon mustard on one side of each chicken cutlet, if desired.

4.Divide the garlic, peppers and Romano cheese between chicken cutlets; roll them up.

5.Bake at 360 degrees F for 25 to 33 minutes until nicely brown on all sides. Serve with the sauerkraut and serve.

Nutrition: 376 Calories; 16.7g Fat; 5.8g Carbs; 47g Protein; 1g Fiber

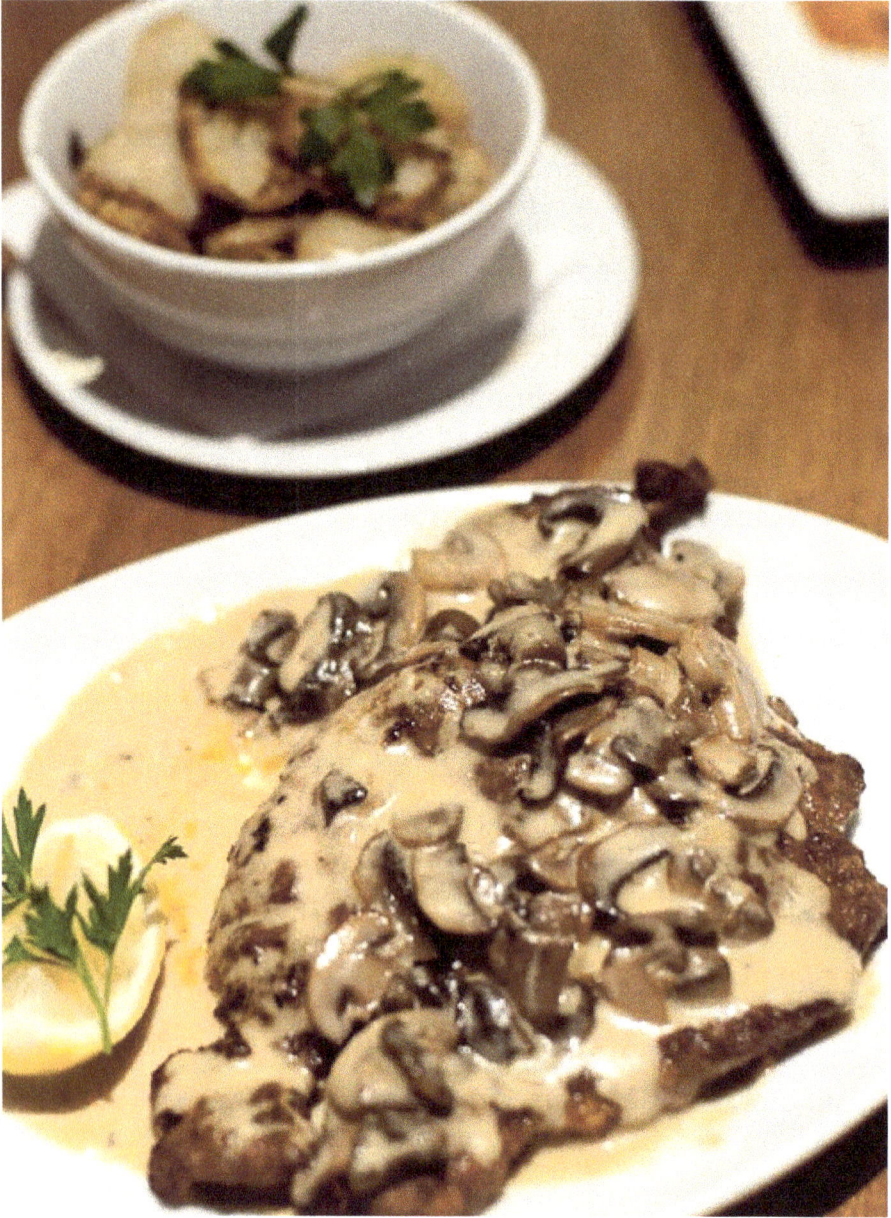

Cream of Chicken Soup

Prep Time:
40 minutes
Serve: 5

Ingredients:

- 1/2 cup Italian peppers, deseeded and chopped
- 1/2 cup green cabbage, shredded
- 5 chicken thighs
- 1/2 cup celery, chopped
- 7 ounces full-fat cream cheese

Directions:

1.Add Italian peppers, cabbage, chicken thighs, and celery to a large clay pot.

2.Pour in 5 cups of water or chicken broth.

3.Partially cover and let it simmer over medium-high heat approximately 30 minutes. Transfer the chicken to a cutting board,

4.Shred the chicken and return it to the pot.

5.Add in full-fat cream cheese and stir until everything is well incorporated.

Nutrition: 514 Calories; 38g Fat; 5.4g Carbs; 35.3g Protein; 0.5g Fiber

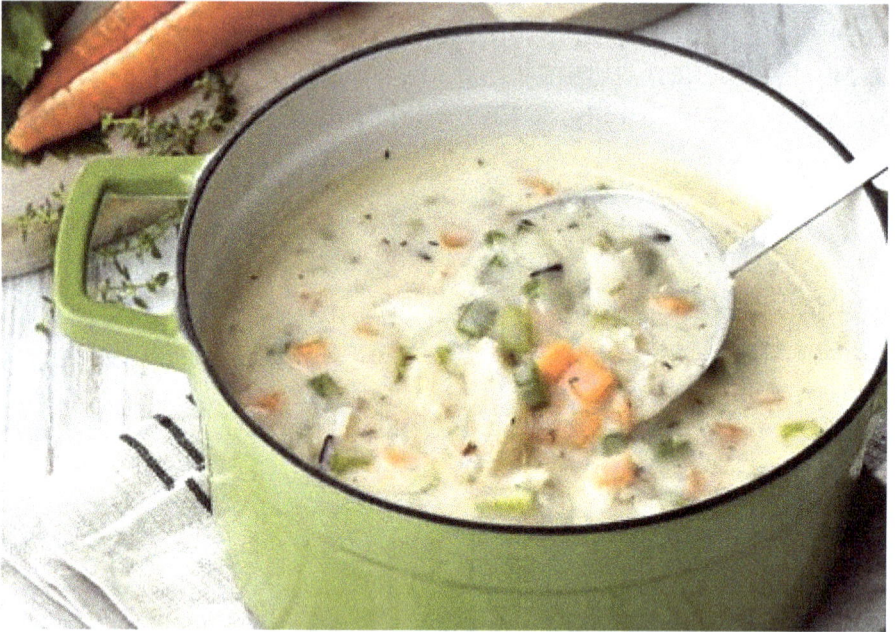

Lemony and Garlicky Chicken Wings

Prep Time:
25 minutes + marinating time
Serve: 4

Ingredients:

- 8 chicken wings
- 2 garlic cloves, minced
- 1/4 cup leeks, chopped
- 2 tablespoons lemon juice
- 1 teaspoon Mediterranean spice mix

Directions:

1.Place all ingredients in a ceramic dish. Cover and let it sit in your refrigerator for 2 hours.

2.Brush the chicken wings with melted ghee. Grill the chicken wings for 15 to 20 minutes, turning them occasionally to ensure even cooking.

Nutrition: 131 Calories; 7.8g Fat; 1.8g Carbs; 13.4g Protein; 0.3g Fiber

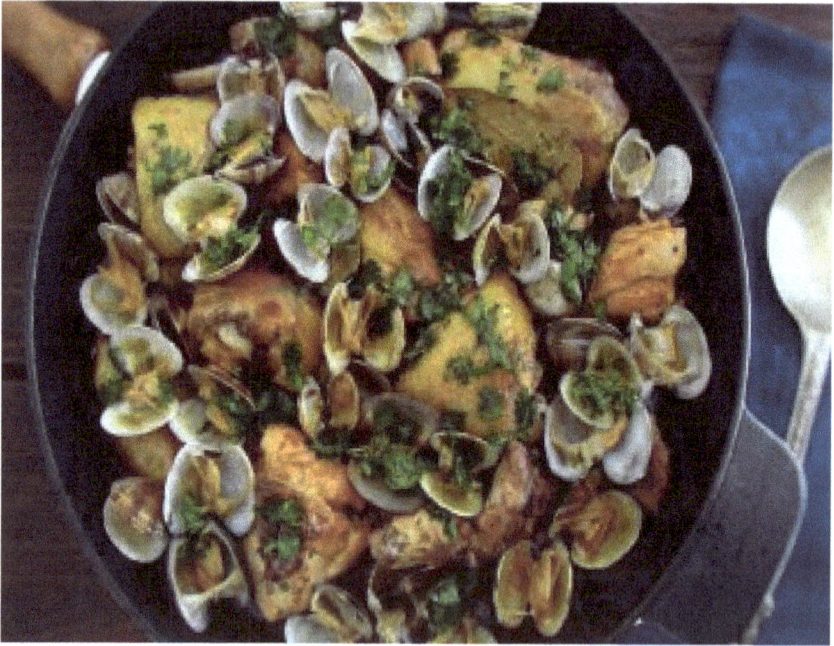

Creamiest Chicken Salad Ever

Prep Time:
1 hour 20 minutes
Serve: 3

Ingredients:

- 1 chicken breast, skinless
- 1/4 mayonnaise
- 1/4 cup sour cream
- 2 tablespoons Cottage cheese, room temperature
- 1/2 avocado, peeled and cubed

Directions:

1.Cook the chicken in a pot of salted water.

2.Remove from the heat and let the chicken sit, covered, in the hot water for 10 to 15 minutes.

3.Slice the chicken into bite-sized strips. Toss with the remaining ingredients.

4.Place in the refrigerator for at least one hour. Serve well chilled.

Nutrition: 400 Calories; 35.1g Fat; 5.6g Carbs; 16.1g Protein; 1g Fiber

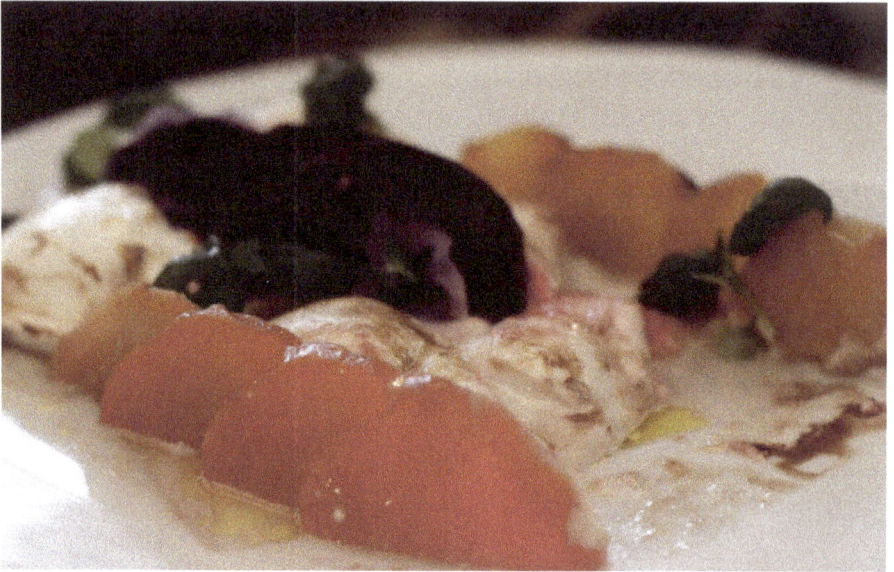

Thai Turkey Curry

Prep Time:
1 hour
Serve: 4

Ingredients:

- 1 pound turkey wings, boneless and chopped
- 2 cloves garlic, finely chopped
- 1 Thai red chili pepper, minced
- 1 cup unsweetened coconut milk, preferably homemade
- 1 cup turkey consommé

Directions:

1.In a saucepan, warm 2 teaspoons of sesame oil. Once hot, brown turkey about 8 minutes or until it is golden brown.

2.Add in the garlic and Thai chili pepper and continue to cook for a minute or so.

3.Add coconut milk and consommé. Season with salt and black pepper to taste.

4.Continue to cook for 40 to 45 minutes over medium heat. Serve warm and enjoy!

Nutrition: 295 Calories; 19.5g Fat; 2.9g Carbs; 25.5g Protein; 1g Fiber

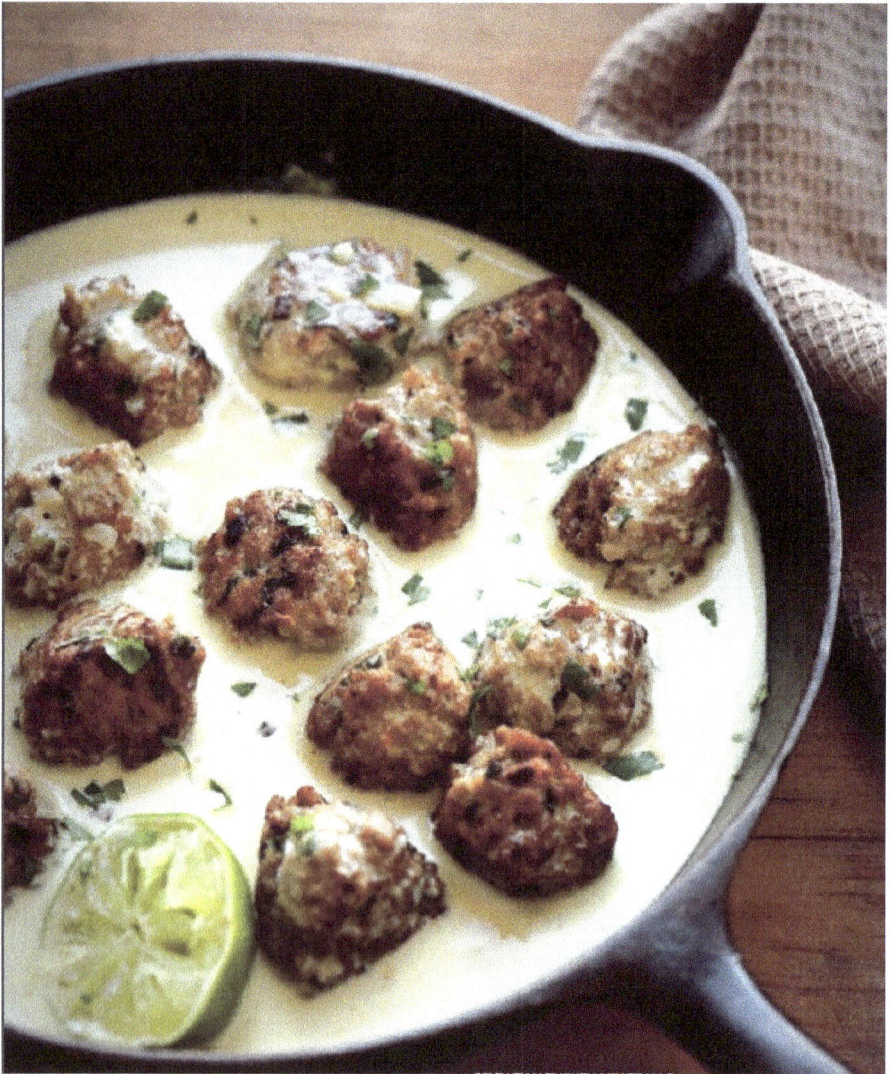

Baked Teriyaki Turkey

Prep Time:
15 minutes
Serve: 2

Ingredients:

- ¾ pound lean ground turkey
- 1 brown onion, chopped
- 1 red bell pepper, deveined and chopped
- 1 serrano pepper, deveined and chopped
- ¼ cup keto teriyaki sauce

Directions:

1.Cook the ground turkey in the preheated pan over medium-high heat; cook for about 5 minutes until no longer pink.

2.Now, sauté the onion and peppers for 3 minutes more.

3.Add in teriyaki sauce and bring the mixture to a boil.

4.Immediately remove from the heat; add in the cooked ground turkey and sautéed mixture.

Nutrition: 410 Calories; 27.1g Fat; 6.6g Carbs; 36.5g Protein; 1g Fiber

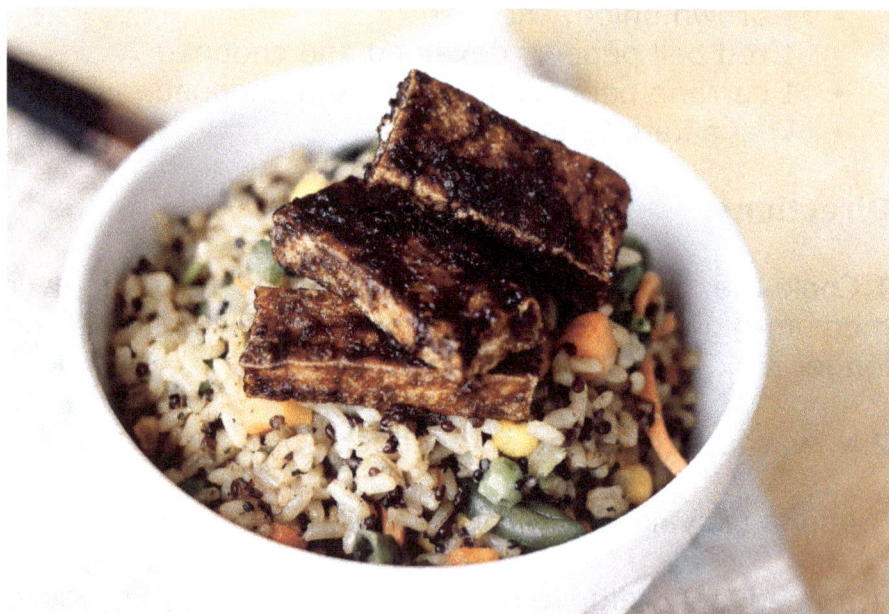

Ranch Turkey with Greek Sauce

Prep Time:
20 minutes
Serve: 4

Ingredients:

- 2 eggs
- 1 tablespoon Ranch seasoning blend
- ½ cup almond meal
- 1 pound turkey tenders,
- 1/2-inch thick
- ½ cup Greek keto sauce

Directions:

1.In a shallow bowl, whisk the eggs with Ranch seasoning blend.

2.In another shallow bowl, place the almond meal. Dip the turkey tenders into the Ranch egg mixture.

3.Then, press them into the almond meal; press to coat well.

4.Heat 2 tablespoons of olive oil in a pan over medium-high heat. Brown turkey tenders for 3 to 4 minutes on each side.

5.Serve the turkey tenders with Greek keto sauce. Enjoy!

Nutrition: 396 Calories; 27.5g Fat; 3.9g Carbs; 33.1g Protein; 1.9g Fiber

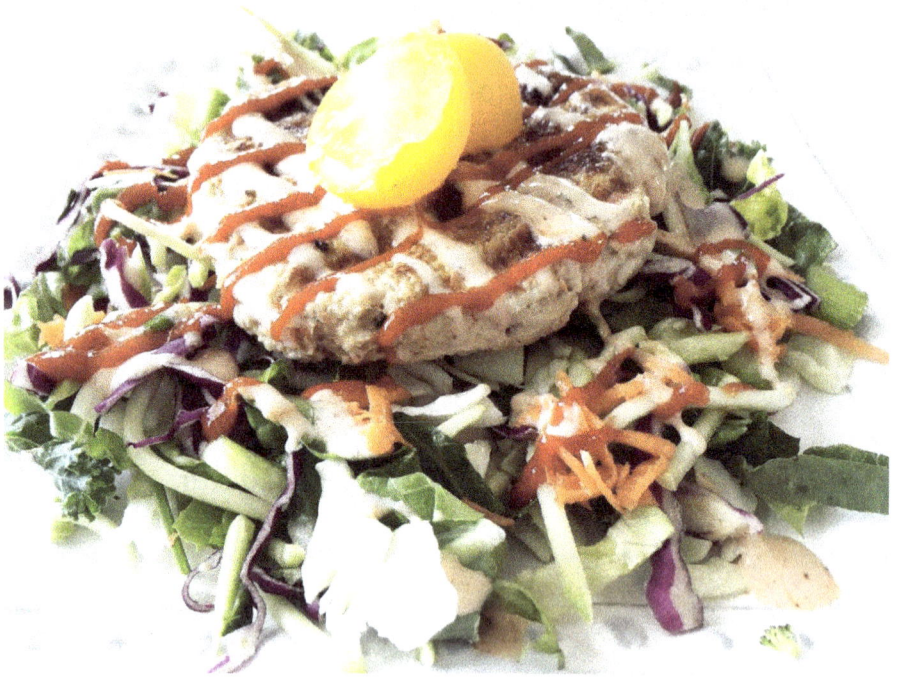

Mediterranean Herbed Chicken

Prep Time:
20 minutes
Serve: 5

Ingredients:

- 2 tablespoons butter, softened at room temperature
- 5 chicken legs, skinless
- 2 scallions, chopped
- 1 tablespoon Mediterranean spice mix
- 1 cup vegetable broth

Directions:

1.In a saucepan, melt 1 tablespoon of butter over a medium-high flame. Now, brown the chicken legs for about 10 minutes, turning them periodically.

2.Add in the remaining tablespoon of butter, scallions, Mediterranean spice mix, and broth.

3.When your mixture reaches boiling, reduce the temperature to a simmer.

4.Continue to simmer for 10 to 11 minutes until cooked through. Taste and adjust the seasoning. Bon appétit!

Nutrition: 370 Calories; 16g Fat; 0.9g Carbs; 51g Protein; 0.2g Fiber

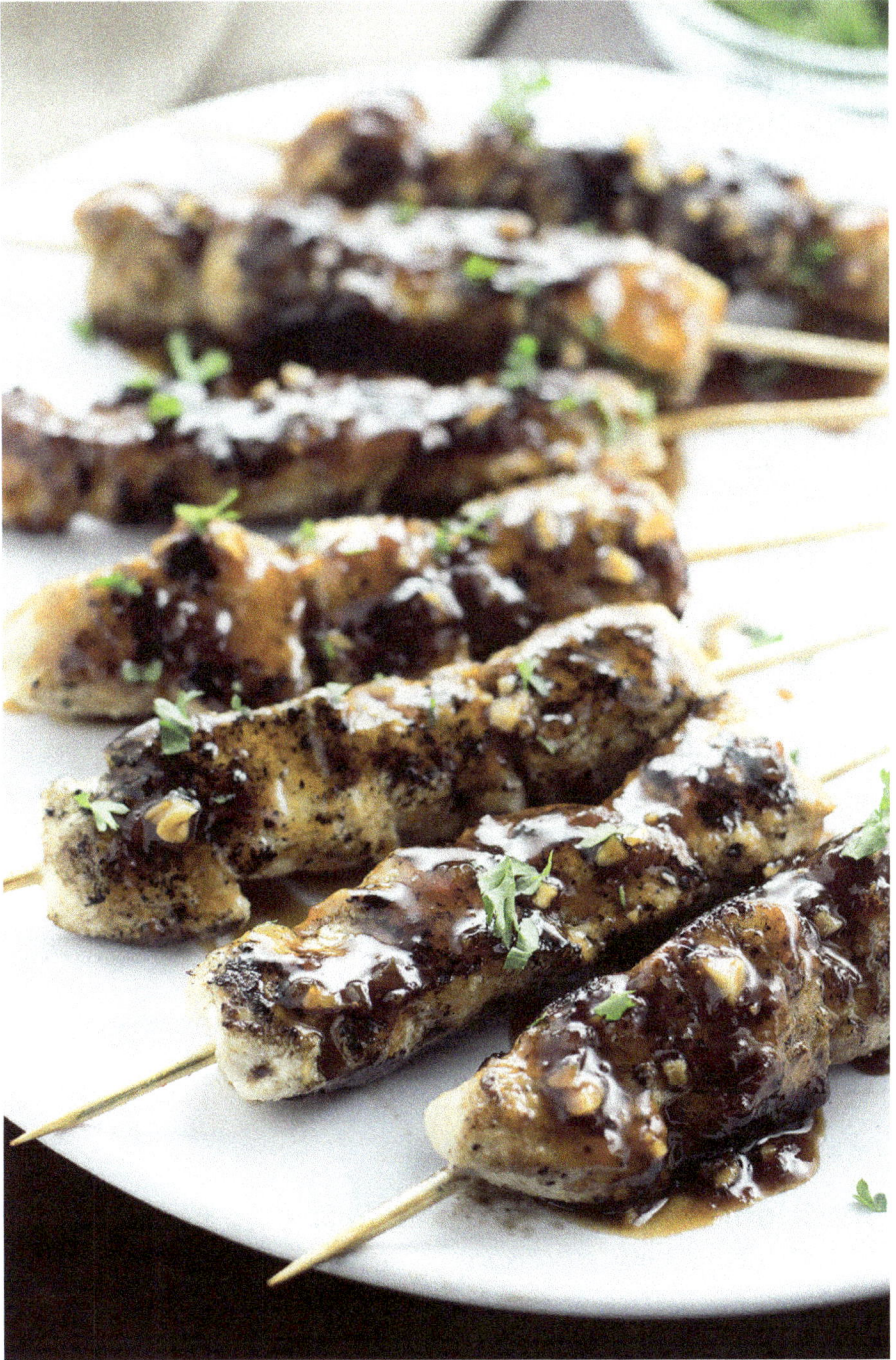

Saucy Chicken with Marsala Wine

Prep Time:
20 minutes
Serve: 2

Ingredients:

- 2 chicken fillets
- 1/4 cup marsala wine
- 1 cup broccoli florets
- 1/4 tomato paste
- 1/2 cup double cream

Directions:

1.Heat 1 tablespoon of olive oil in a sauté pan over medium-high heat. Once hot, sear the chicken for 10 minutes, flipping them over once or twice.

2.Add marsala wine and deglaze the pot. Add in the broccoli and tomato paste.

3.Reduce the heat to simmer.

4.Continue to simmer for a further 5 to 7 minutes. Lastly, stir in the double cream. Season with paprika, salt, and black pepper to taste.

Nutrition: 347 Calories; 20.4g Fat; 4.7g Carbs; 35.3g Protein; 1.4g Fiber

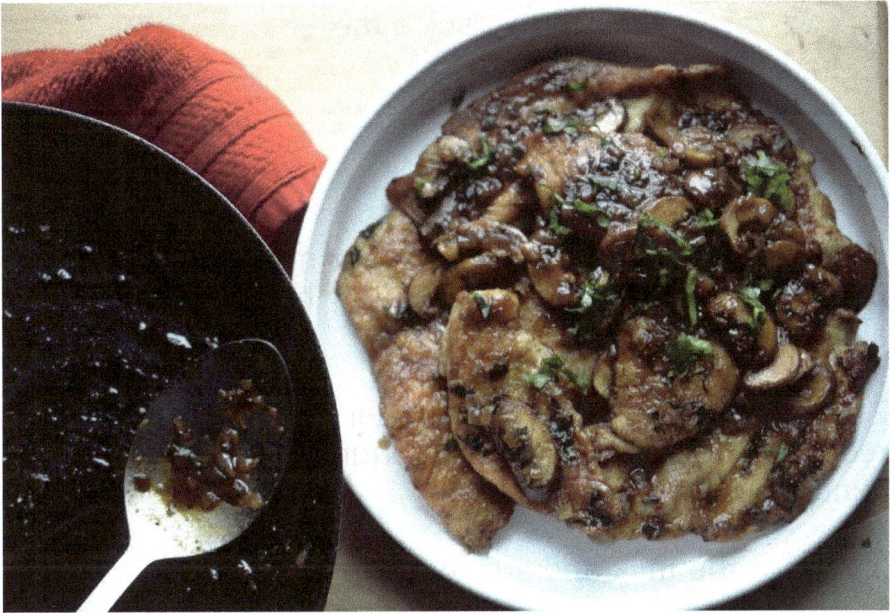

Chicken Mulligatawny

Prep Time:
35 minutes
Serve: 4

Ingredients:

- 2 tablespoons ghee
- 1 pound chicken thighs, boneless and skinless
- 1 tablespoon Indian spice mix
- 1 celery stalk, chopped
- 1 cup milk

Directions:

1.Melt the butter in a soup pot over medium-high flame. Brown the chicken thighs until nicely browned on all sides about 6 minutes.

2.Add in Indian spice mix and celery; stir to combine and reduce the heat to simmer; continue to simmer for 30 minutes more.

3.Pour in the milk and stir to combine well. Bon appétit!

Nutrition: 343 Calories; 26.7g Fat; 3.8g Carbs; 20.9g Protein; 0.2g Fiber

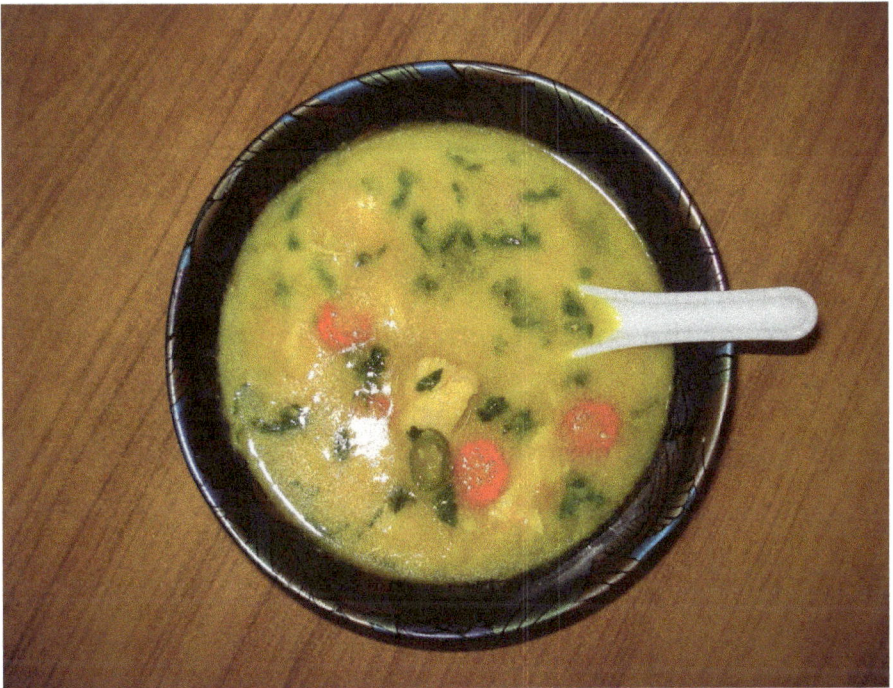

Naga Chicken Salad Ole

Prep Time:
20 minutes + chilling time
Serve: 6

Ingredients:

- 1/2 cup dry white wine
- 1 ½ pounds chicken breasts
- 1 Spanish naga chili pepper, chopped
- 1/4 cup mayonnaise
- 2 cups arugula

Directions:

1.Place the chicken breasts and wine in a deep saucepan. Then, cover the chicken with water, and bring to a boil.

2.When your mixture reaches boiling, reduce the temperature to a simmer.

3.Let it simmer, partially covered, for about 13 minutes or until cooked through.

4.Shred the chicken, discarding the bones and poaching liquid.

5.Place in a salad bowl and add naga chili pepper, arugula, and mayonnaise to the bowl.

6.Add Spanish peppers, if desired and stir to combine well.

Nutrition: 278 Calories; 16.1g Fat; 4.9g Carbs; 27.2g Protein; 0.9g Fiber

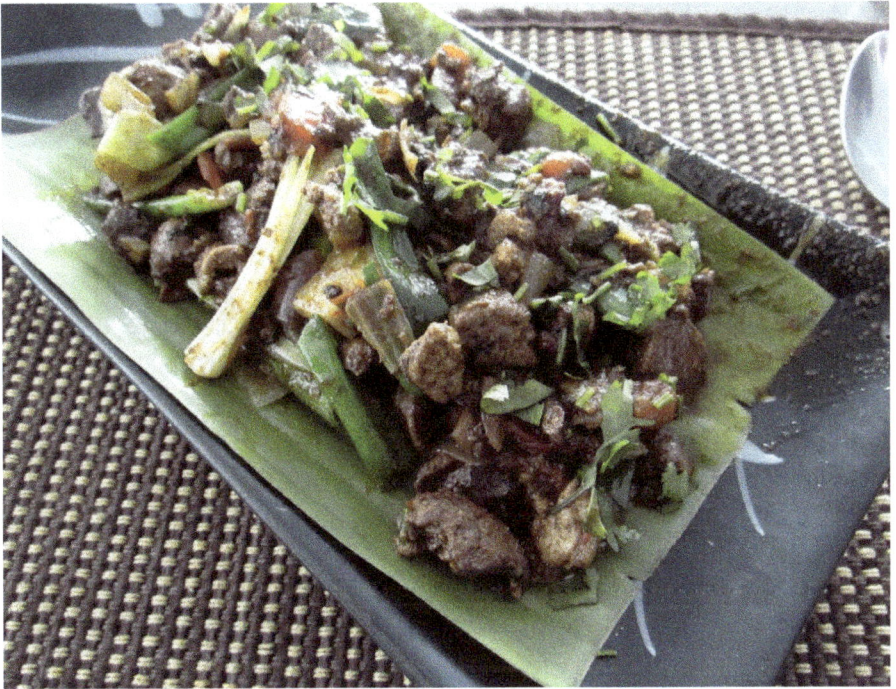

Oven-Roasted Chimichurri Chicken

Prep Time:
40 minutes + marinating time
Serve: 5

Ingredients:

- 1 ½ pounds chicken tenders
- ½ cup fresh parsley, chopped
- 2 garlic cloves, minced
- ¼ cup olive oil
- 4 tablespoons white wine vinegar

Directions:

1.Blend the parsley, olive oil, vinegar, and garlic in your food processor until the smooth and uniform sauce forms. Pierce the chicken with a small knife.

2.Add chicken and 1/2 of the chimichurri sauce to a glass dosh and let them marinate for 2 hours in your refrigerator.

3.Spritz a baking pan with nonstick cooking spray. Place the chicken in the baking pan. Season with salt and black pepper.

4.Bake in the preheated oven at 360 degrees F for 35 minutes or until an internal temperature reaches about 165 degrees F.

5.Serve with the reserved chimichurri sauce. Bon appétit!

Nutrition: 305 Calories; 14.7g Fat; 0.8g Carbs; 27.9g Protein; 0.2g Fiber

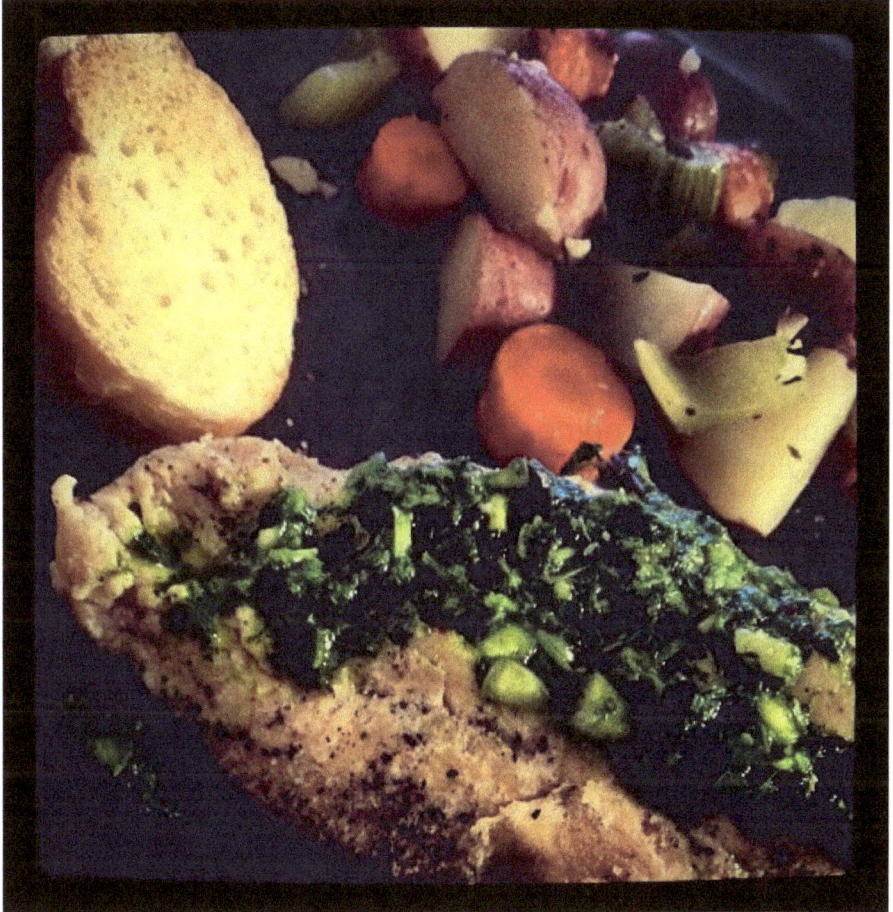

Classic Garlicky Chicken Drumettes

Prep Time:
40 minutes + marinating time
Serve: 5

Ingredients:

- ¼ cup coconut aminos
- 1 tablespoon olive oil
- 1 tablespoon apple cider vinegar
- 2 cloves garlic, minced
- 5 chicken drumettes

Directions:

1.Thoroughly combine, coconut aminos, olive oil, apple cider vinegar, and garlic in a glass dish.

2.Allow it to marinate for 2 hours in your refrigerator

3.Place the chicken in a foil-lined baking dish. Season with salt and black pepper to taste.

4.Bake in the preheated oven at 410 degrees F for 35 minutes, basting the chicken with the reserved marinade.

Nutrition: 266 Calories; 19.3g Fat; 0.8g Carbs; 20.3g Protein; 0.2g Fiber

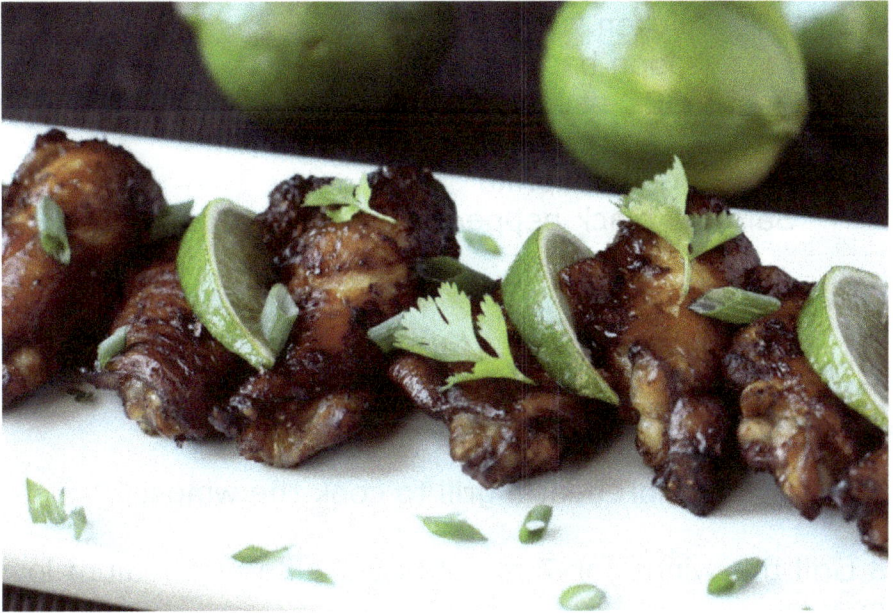

Barbeque Chicken Wings

Prep Time:
15 minutes
Cook Time:
14 minutes
Serve: 6

Ingredients:

- 2 lb. chicken wings
- ½ teaspoon basil; dried
- ¾ cup BBQ sauce
- 1 teaspoon red pepper; crushed.
- 2 teaspoons paprika
- Salt and black pepper to the taste

Directions:

1.Start by tossing the chicken wings with remaining ingredients in a bowl.

2.Prepare and preheat a grill to cook the wings.

3.Grill the wings for 7 minutes per side on medium low heat.

Nutrition: Calories 251, Total Fat 15.3 g, Saturated Fat 6.5 g, Cholesterol 122 mg, Sodium 366 mg, Total Carbs 3 g, Fiber 1.8 g, Sugar 0.9 g, Protein 25 g

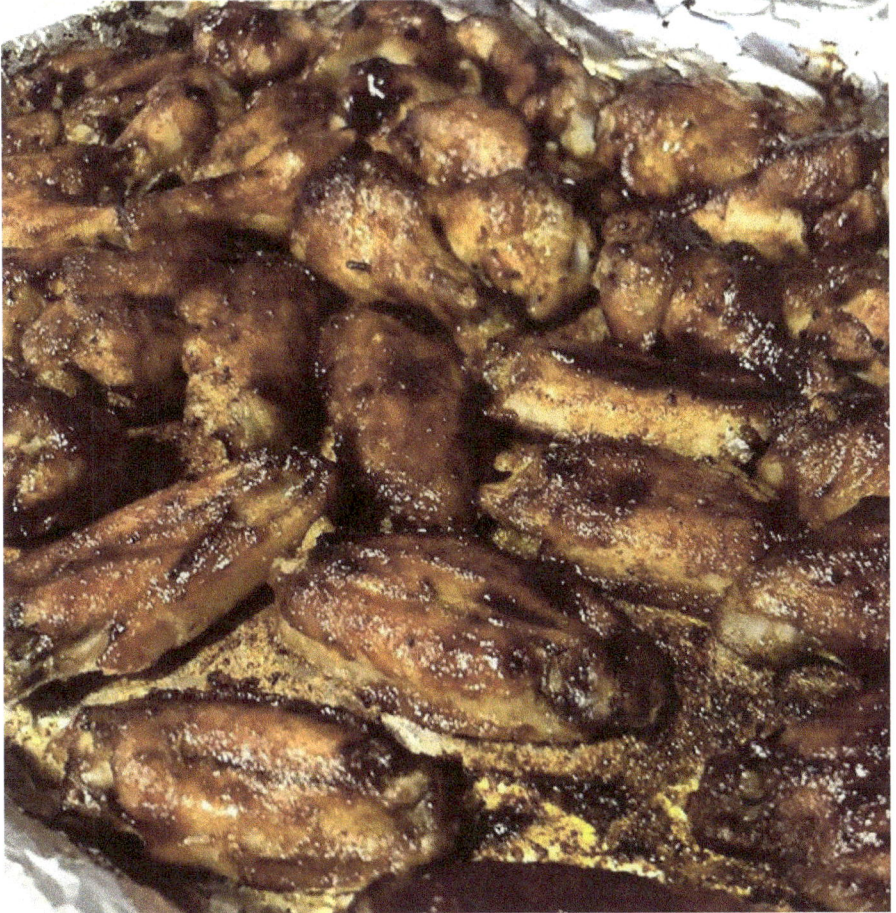

Saucy Duck

Prep Time:
15 minutes
Cook Time:
15 minutes
Serve: 2

Ingredients:

- 1 duck, cut into small chunks
- 2 tablespoon ginger garlic paste
- 2 green onions; roughly chopped
- 4 tablespoon soy sauce
- 4 tablespoon sherry wine
- Salt and black pepper to the taste

Directions:

1.Start by tossing the duck with all other ingredients in a bowl.

2.Marinate the meat for 4 hours in the refrigerator.

3.Spread the duck chunks in a baking tray.

4.Bake the meat for 15 minutes with occasional tossing.

Nutrition: Calories 225, Total Fat 14.3 g, Saturated Fat 0.6 g, Cholesterol 137 mg, Sodium 538 mg, Total Carbs 2.8 g, Fiber 7 g, Sugar 0.3 g, Protein 28.2 g

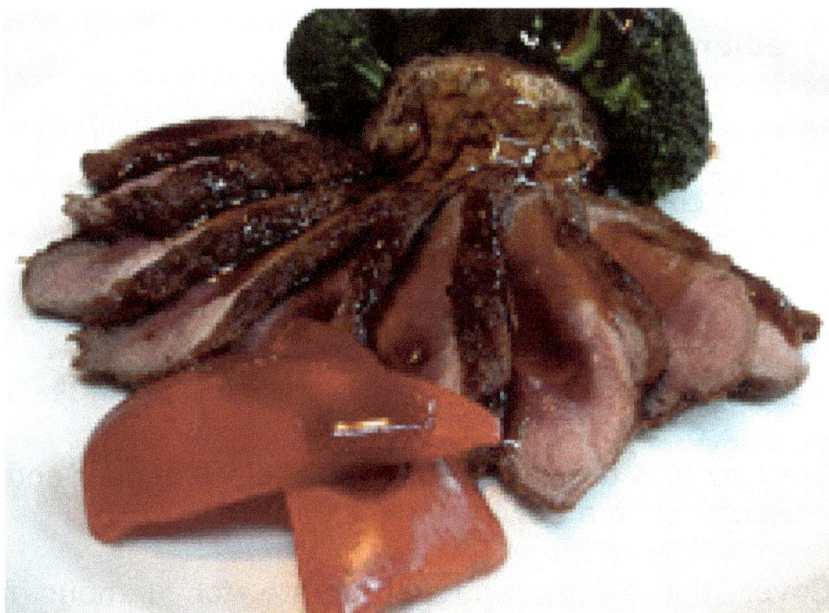

Chicken Roux Gumbo

Prep Time:
15 minutes
Cook Time:
20 minutes
Serve: 2

Ingredients:

- 1 lb. chicken thighs; cut into halves
- ¼ cup 1 tablespoon vegetable oil
- 1/2 cup almond flour
- 1 cup vegetable stock
- 1 teaspoon Cajun spice
- Salt and black pepper to the taste

Directions:

1.Start by toss the chicken with salt, black pepper and 1 tablespoon oil in a bowl.

2.Cover the thighs and refrigerate for 1 hour for marination.

3.Sear the marinated chicken in a sauté pan.

4.Cook for 5 minutes per side until golden brown.

5.Whisk almond flour with Cajun spice and remaining oil in a separate bowl.

6.Add almond mixture to a cooking pot and stir cook for 2 minutes.

7.Stir in stock and cook well until it thickens.

8.Toss in the sear chicken and cook for 4 minutes.

Nutrition: Calories 433, Total Fat 15.2 g, Saturated Fat 8.6 g, Cholesterol 179 mg, Sodium 318 mg, Total Carbs 2.7 g, Fiber 1.1 g, Sugar 1.1 g, Protein 68.4 g

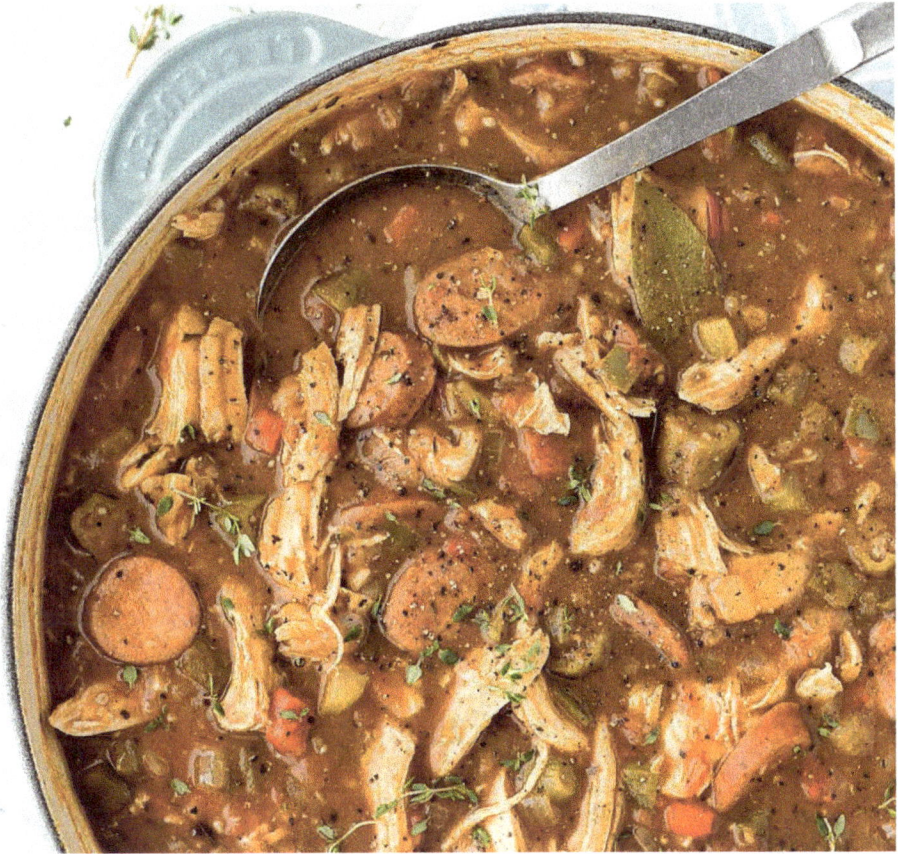

Chunky Salsa Chicken

Prep Time:
15 minutes
Cook Time:
25 minutes
Serve: 2

Ingredients:

- 1 lb. chicken breast, skinless and boneless
- 1 cup chunky salsa
- ¾ teaspoon cumin
- A pinch of oregano
- Salt and black pepper to the taste

Directions:

1. Pat dry the chicken and rub it with salt and pepper.

2. Place this chicken in the insert of the Instant Pot.

3. Add cumin, oregano and chunky salsa.

4. Mix well then seal the lid of the Instant Pot.

5. Cook on poultry mode for 25 minutes.

6. Once done, release the pressure quickly then shred meat with a fork.

7. Serve the meat with its salsa.

Nutrition: Calories 272, Total Fat 27 g, Saturated Fat 16 g, Cholesterol 83 mg, Sodium 175 mg, Total Carbs 7.8 g, Fiber 0.4 g, Sugar 5.2 g, Protein 5.3 g

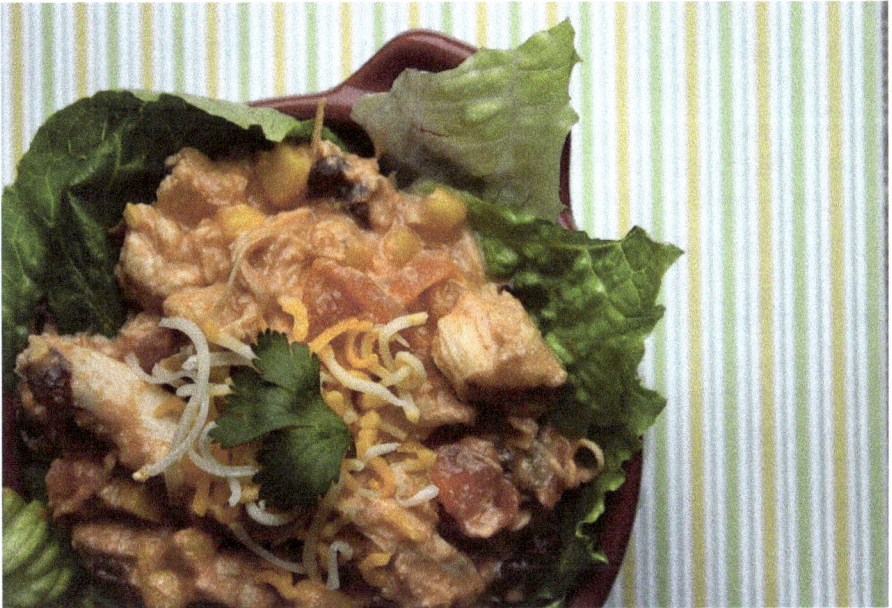

Dijon Chicken

Prep Time:
 15 minutes
Cook Time:
20 minutes
Serve: 6

Ingredients:

- 2 lb. chicken thighs; skinless and boneless
- 1/4 cup lemon juice
- 2 tablespoon extra-virgin olive oil
- 3 tablespoon Dijon mustard
- 2 tablespoon Italian seasoning
- Salt and black pepper to the taste

Directions:

1.Start by tossing chicken with all other ingredients in a bowl.

2.Prepare and preheat the grill on medium heat.

3.Grill the chicken pieces for 5 minutes per side until al dente.

Nutrition: Calories 242, Total Fat 15.9 g, Saturated Fat 10.6 g, Cholesterol 36 mg, Sodium 421 mg, Total Carbs 4.6 g, Fiber 2 g, Sugar 1.6 g, Protein 20.8 g

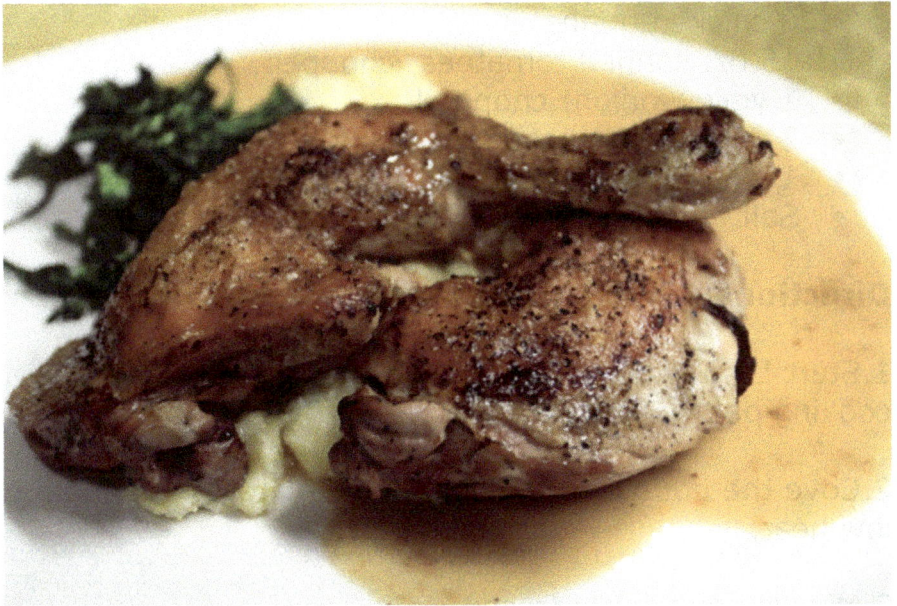

Chicken Thighs with Vegetables

Prep Time:
15 minutes
Cook Time:
30 minutes
Serve: 6

Ingredients:

- 6 chicken thighs
- 15 oz. canned tomatoes; chopped.
- 1 yellow onion; chopped.
- 2 cups chicken stock
- 1/4 lb. baby carrots; cut into halves
- Salt and black pepper to the taste

Directions:

1.Start by adding chicken and all other ingredients to a cooking pot.

2.Cove the pot's lid and cook for 30 minutes on medium low heat.

3.Mix well and serve fresh.

Nutrition: Calories 362, Total Fat 15.9 g, Saturated Fat 9.9 g, Cholesterol 49 mg, Sodium 684 mg, Total Carbs 4.1 g, Fiber 1.4 g, Sugar 1.1 g, Protein 23.3 g

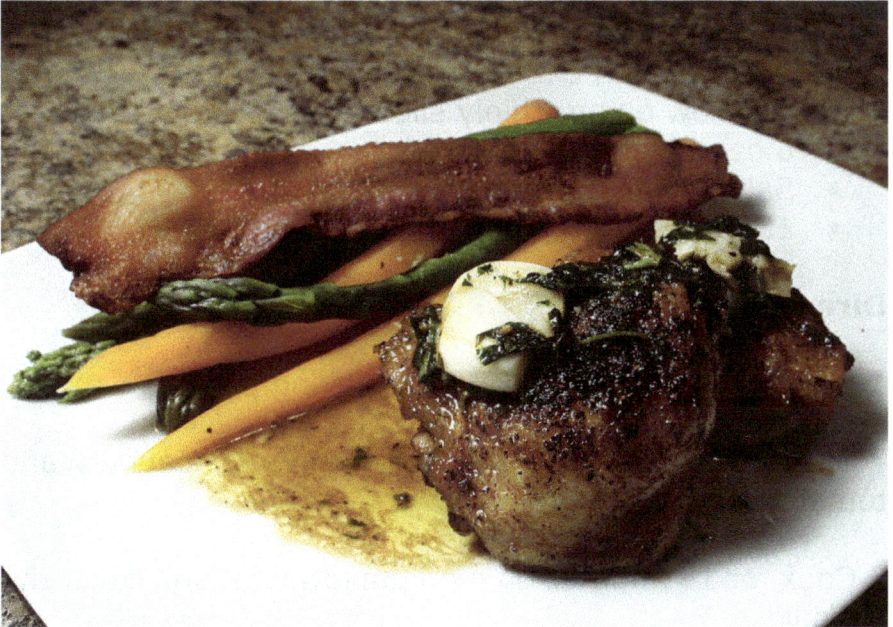

Chicken Dipped in Tomatillo Sauce

Prep Time:
15 minutes
Cook Time:
15 minutes
Serve: 2

Ingredients:

- 1 lb. chicken thighs; skinless and boneless
- 2 tablespoon extra-virgin olive oil
- 1 yellow onion; thinly sliced
- 5 oz. tomatoes; chopped.
- Salt and black pepper to the taste
- 15 oz. canned tomatillos; chopped.

Directions:

1.Start by heating olive oil in a cooking pot.

2.Toss in chicken, tomatillos, onion, salt, pepper, and tomatoes.

3.Cook for 15 minutes on medium low heat and cover the pot's lid.

4.Stir well and serve fresh.

Nutrition: Calories 260, Total Fat 13 g, Saturated Fat 5 g, Cholesterol 0.3 mg, Sodium 465 mg, Total Carbs 6 g, Fiber 5.4 g, Sugar 1.3 g, Protein 26 g

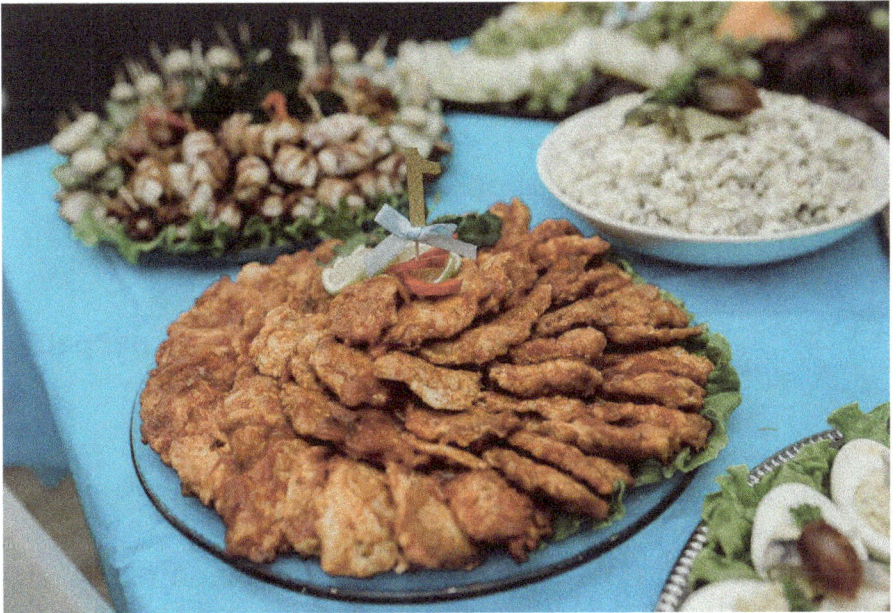

Crispy Italian Chicken

Prep Time:
15 minutes
Cook Time:
10 minutes
Serve: 6

Ingredients:

- 6 chicken thighs
- 1 cup almond flour
- 2 eggs; whisked
- 1 ½ cups panko breadcrumbs
- Salt and black pepper to the taste

Directions:

1.Start by tossing the flour with salt and black pepper in a flat plate.

2.Whisk the eggs in a separate bowl and spread breadcrumbs in a plate.

3.Coat the chicken thighs with the flour then dip in the eggs and then coat with crumbs.

4.Prepare and preheat the grill on medium heat.

5.Grill the chicken for 5 minutes per side on medium heat.

Nutrition: Calories 355, Total Fat 16.8 g, Saturated Fat 4 g, Cholesterol 150 mg, Sodium 719 mg, Total Carbs 1.4 g, Fiber 0.5 g, Sugar 0.1 g, Protein 47 g

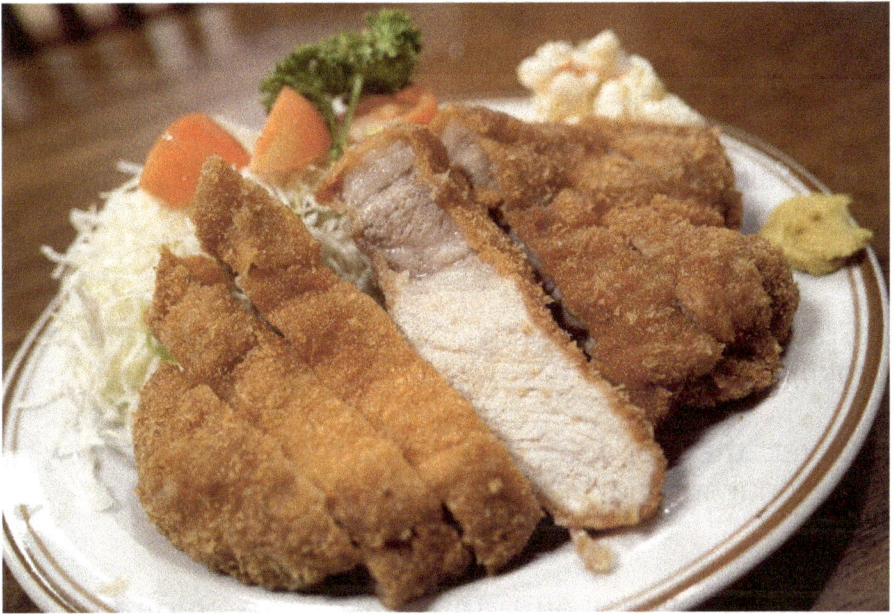

Cacciatore Olive Chicken

Prep Time:
15 minutes
Cook Time:
20 minutes
Serve: 8

Ingredients:

- 28 oz. canned tomatoes and juice; crushed.
- 8 chicken drumsticks; bone-in
- ½ cup olives; pitted and sliced
- 1 cup chicken stock
- 1 yellow onion; chopped.
- Salt and black pepper, to the taste

Directions:

1.Start by adding chicken and all other ingredients to a cooking pot.

2.Cover the pot's lid and cook for 20 minutes with occasional stirring.

Nutrition: Calories 489, Total Fat 18.7 g, Saturated Fat 3.8 g, Cholesterol 151 mg, Sodium 636 mg, Total Carbs 6.1 g, Fiber 0.5 g, Sugar 4.3 g, Protein 50 g

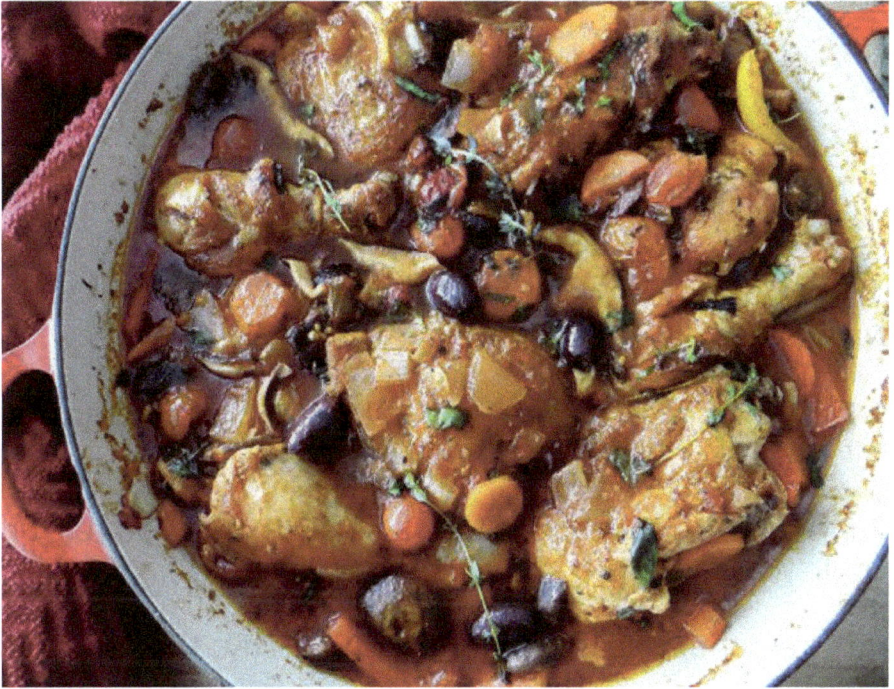

Duck and Vegetable Stew

Prep Time:
15 minutes
Cook Time:
40 minutes
Serve: 6

Ingredients:

- 1 duck; chopped into medium pieces
- 2 carrots; chopped
- 2 cups of water
- 1 cucumber; chopped
- 1-inch ginger pieces; chopped
- Salt and black pepper to the taste

Directions:

1.Place the duck pieces in the Instant Pot Add carrots, wine, ginger, water, salt, and pepper.

2.Mix well and seal the lid. Cook for 40 minutes on Poultry mode.

3.Once done, release the pressure quickly, then remove the lid.

Nutrition: Calories 325, Total Fat 14.4 g, Saturated Fat 3.5 g, Cholesterol 135 mg, Sodium 552 mg, Total Carbs 2.3 g, Fiber 0.4 g, Sugar 0.5 g, Protein 44 g

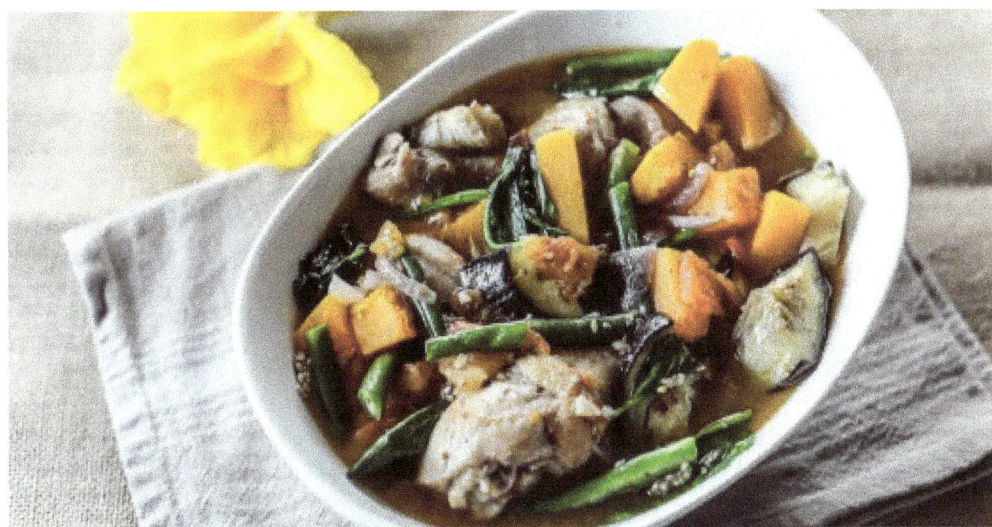

Chicken Eggplant Curry

Prep Time:
15 minutes
Cook Time:
15 minutes
Serve: 4

Ingredients:

- 8 chicken pieces
- 1 eggplant; cubed
- 3 garlic cloves; crushed.
- 14 oz. canned coconut milk
- 2 tablespoon green curry paste
- Salt and black pepper to the taste

Directions:

1.Start by adding chicken and all other ingredients to a cooking pot.

2.Cover the pot's lid and cook for 15 minutes with occasional stirring.

Nutrition: Calories 452, Total Fat 3.5 g, Saturated Fat 0.5 g, Cholesterol 181 mg, Sodium 461 mg, Total Carbs 7.5 g, Fiber 1.7 g, Sugar 1.3 g, Protein 91.8 g

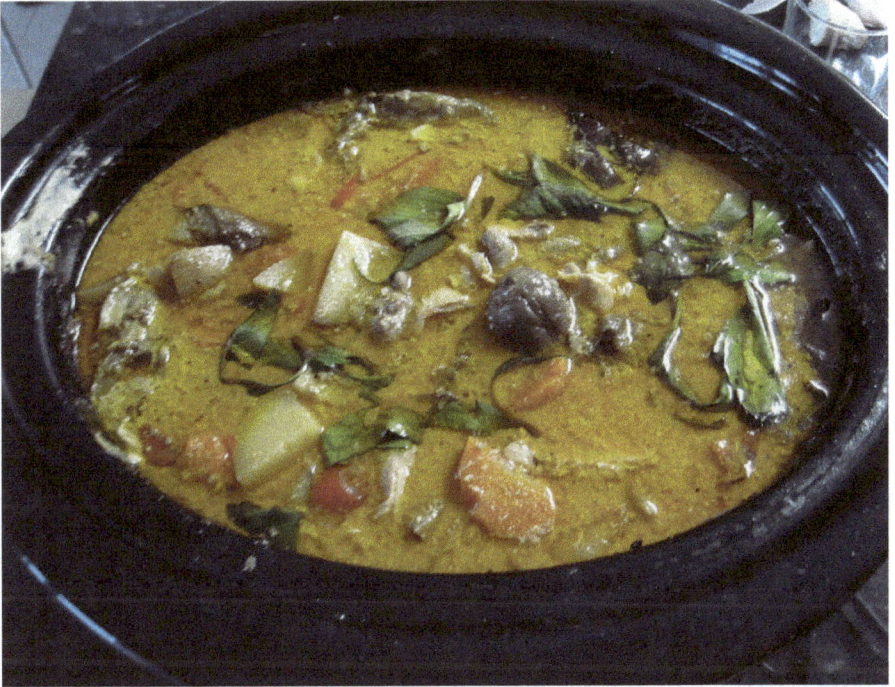

Mushroom Cream Goose Curry

Prep Time:
15 minutes
Cook Time:
25 minutes
Serve: 4

Ingredients:

- 12 oz. canned mushroom cream
- 3 goose breasts; fat trimmed off and cut into pieces
- 1 yellow onion; chopped.
- 3 ½ cups water
- 2 teaspoon garlic; minced.
- Salt and black pepper to the taste

Directions:

1.Start by adding chicken and all other ingredients to a cooking pot.

2.Cover the pot's lid and cook for 25 minutes with occasional stirring.

Nutrition: Calories 386, Total Fat 10 g, Saturated Fat 1.7 g, Cholesterol 93 mg, Sodium 179 mg, Total Carbs 11.7 g, Fiber 0.4 g, Sugar 0.7 g, Protein 25.7 g

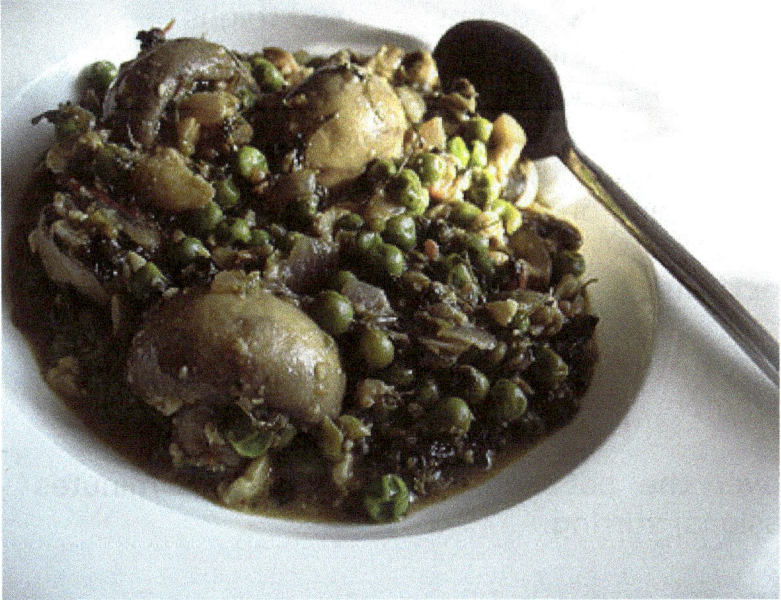

Chicken Curry

Prep Time:
15 minutes
Cook Time:
25 minutes
Serve: 8

Ingredients:

- 3 lb. chicken drumsticks and thighs
- 1 yellow onion; finely chopped
- 1 cup chicken stock
- 15 oz. canned tomatoes; crushed.
- 1 lb. spinach; chopped.
- Salt and black pepper to the taste

Directions:

1.Start by adding chicken and all other ingredients to a cooking pot.

2.Cover the pot's lid and cook for 25 minutes with occasional stirring.

Nutrition: Calories 283, Total Fat 23 g, Saturated Fat 7.9 g, Cholesterol 69 mg, Sodium 106 mg, Total Carbs 0.2 g, Fiber 0.1 g, Sugar 0 g, Protein 18 g

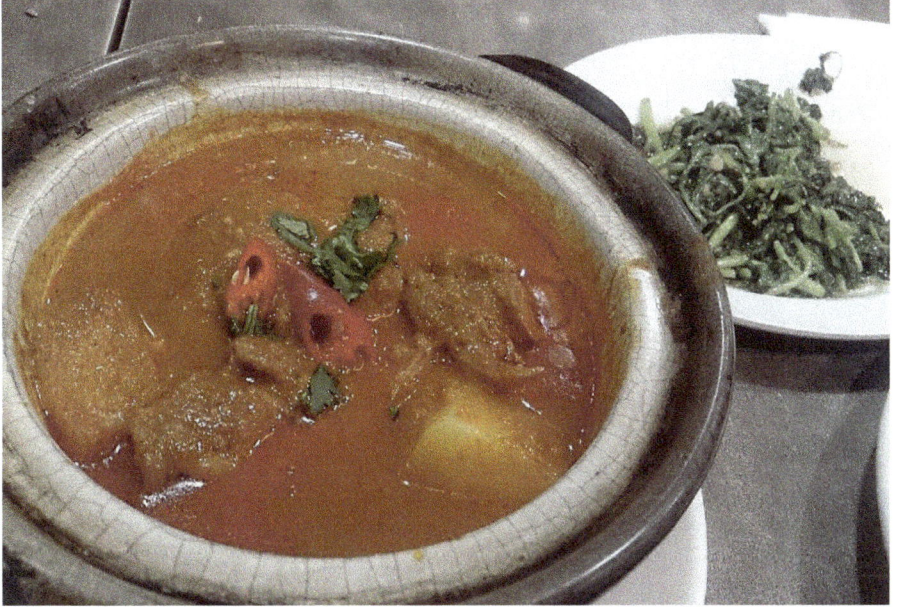

Saucy Teriyaki Chicken

Prep Time:
15 minutes
Cook Time:
25 minutes
Serve: 4

Ingredients:

- 2 lb. chicken breasts; skinless and boneless, diced
- 1 cup teriyaki sauce
- ½ cup chicken stock
- A handful green onions; chopped.
- Salt and black pepper to the taste

Directions:

1.Start by adding chicken and all other ingredients to a cooking pot.

2.Cover the pot's lid and cook for 25 minutes with occasional stirring.

Nutrition: Calories 402, Total Fat 20.8 g, Saturated Fat 5 g, Cholesterol 130 mg, Sodium 112 mg, Total Carbs 2.9 g, Fiber 0.9 g, Sugar 0.8 g, Protein 50.5 g

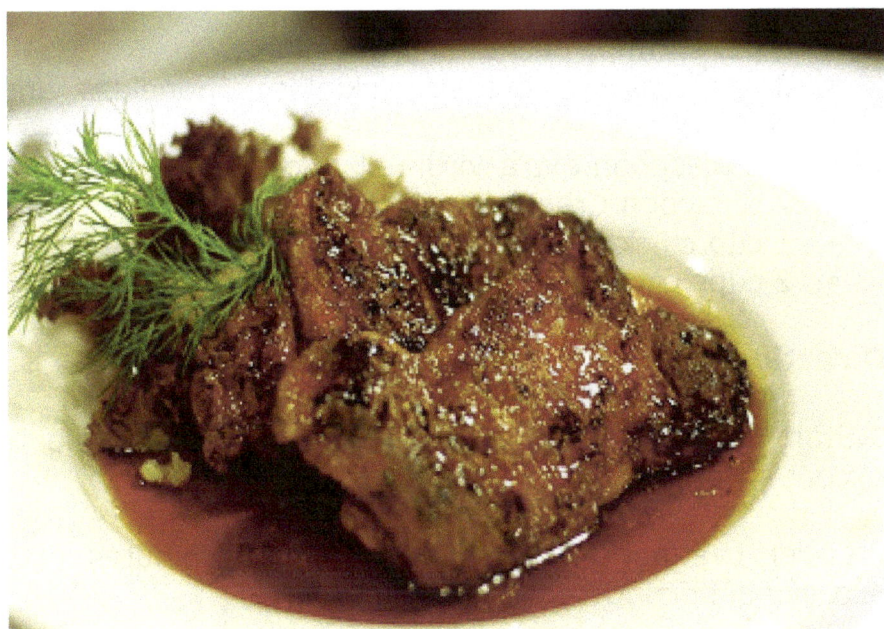

Chicken Shrimp Curry

Prep Time:
15 minutes
Cook Time:
20 minutes
Serve: 2

Ingredients:

- 8 oz. shrimp; peeled and deveined
- 8 oz. chicken breasts; skinless; boneless and chopped.
- 2 tablespoon extra-virgin olive oil
- 2 teaspoon Creole seasoning
- 1 cup chicken stock
- 2 cups canned tomatoes; chopped.

Directions:

1.Start by adding chicken and all other ingredients except shrimp to a cooking pot.

2.Cover the pot's lid and cook for 15 minutes with occasional stirring.

3.Toss in shrimp and cook for another 5 minutes.

Nutrition: Calories 377, Total Fat 11.4 g, Saturated Fat 1.8 g, Cholesterol 168 mg, Sodium 215 mg, Total Carbs 10.4 g, Fiber 0.2 g, Sugar 0.1 g, Protein 64 g

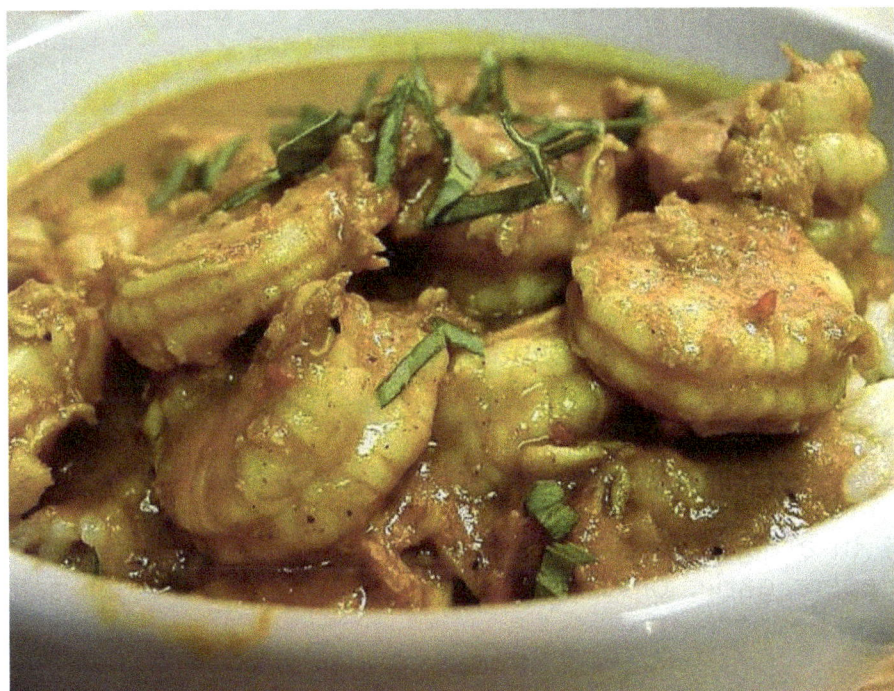

Whole Chicken with Prunes and Capers

Prep Time:
55 minutes
Serve: 6

Ingredients:

- 1 whole chicken, 3 lb
- ½ cup pitted prunes
- 3 minced cloves of garlic
- 2 tbsp capers
- 2 bay leaves
- 2 tbsp red wine vinegar
- 2 tbsp olive oil
- 1 tbsp dried oregano
- ¼ cup packed brown sugar
- 1 tbsp chopped and fresh parsley
- Salt and black pepper

Directions:

1.In a big and deep bowl, mix the prunes, the olives, capers, garlic, olive oil, bay leaves, oregano, vinegar, salt and pepper.

2.Spread the mixture on the bottom of a baking tray, and place the chicken.

3.Preheat the Air Fryer to 360 F. Sprinkle a little bit of brown sugar on top of the chicken; cook for 55 minutes.

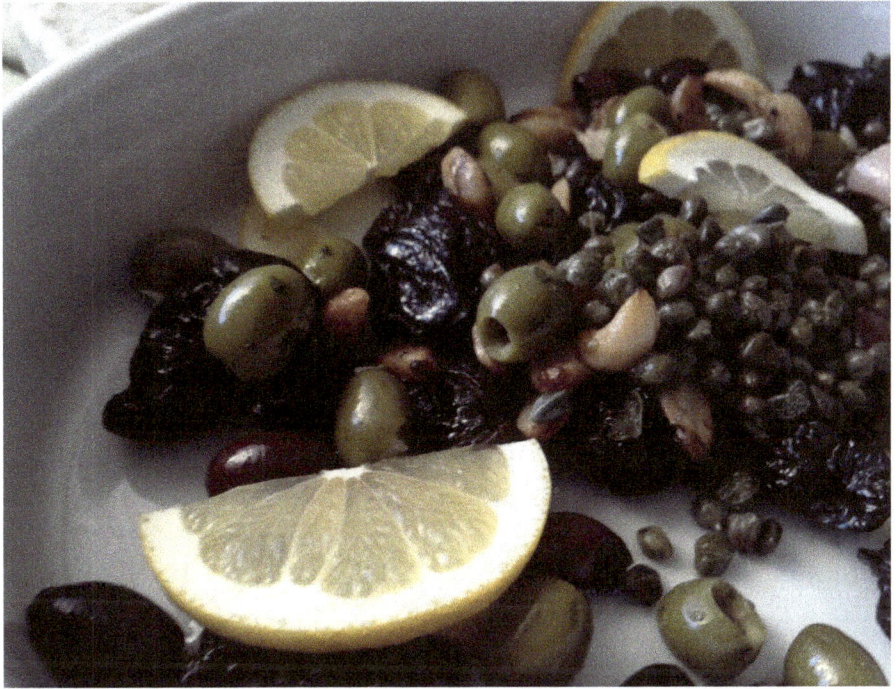

White Wine Chicken with Herbs

Prep Time:
45 minutes
Serve: 6

Ingredients:

- 1 whole chicken, around 3 lb, cut in pieces
- 3 chopped cloves of garlic
- ½ cup olive oil
- ½ cup white wine
- 1 tbsp fresh rosemary
- 1 tbsp chopped fresh oregano
- 1 tbsp fresh thyme
- Juice from 1 lemon
- Salt and black pepper, to taste

Directions:

1.In a large bowl, combine cloves of garlic, rosemary, thyme, olive oil, lemon juice, oregano, salt and pepper.

2.Mix all ingredients very well and spread the mixture into a baking dish. Add the chicken and stir.

3.Preheat the Air Fryer to 380 F, and transfer in the chicken mixture. Sprinkle with wine and cook for 45 minutes.

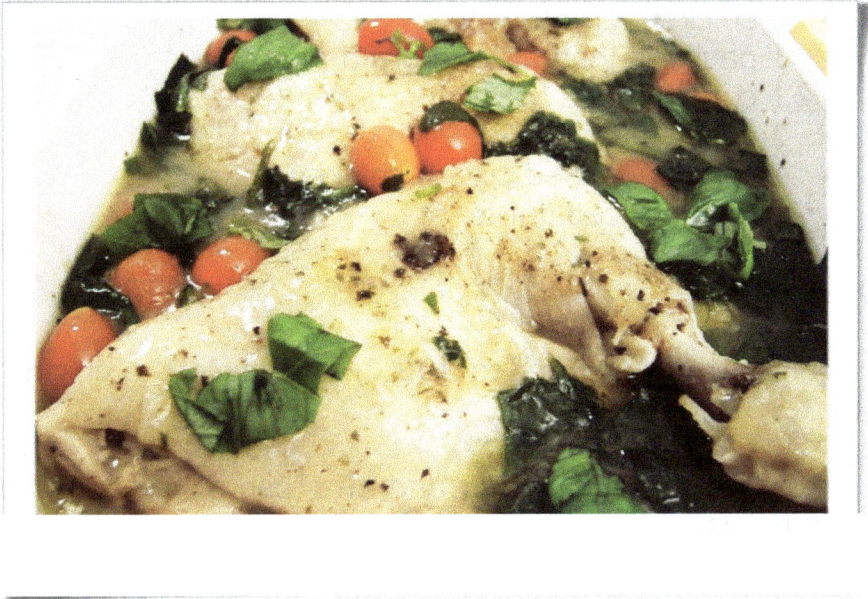

Tasty Chicken Quarters with Broccoli & Rice

Prep Time:
60 minutes
Serve: 3

Ingredients:

- 3 chicken leg quarters
- 1 package instant long grain rice
- 1 cup chopped broccoli
- 2 cups water
- 1 can condensed cream chicken soup
- 1 tbsp minced garlic

Directions:

1.Preheat the Air Fryer to 390 F, and place the chicken quarters in the Air Fryer.

2.Season with salt, pepper and one tbsp of oil; cook for 30 minutes.

3.Meanwhile, in a large deep bowl, mix the rice, water, minced garlic, soup and broccoli. Combine the mixture very well.

4.Remove the chicken from the Air fryer and place it on a platter to drain.

5.Spread the rice mixture on the bottom of the dish and place the chicken on top of the rice. Cook again for 30 minutes.

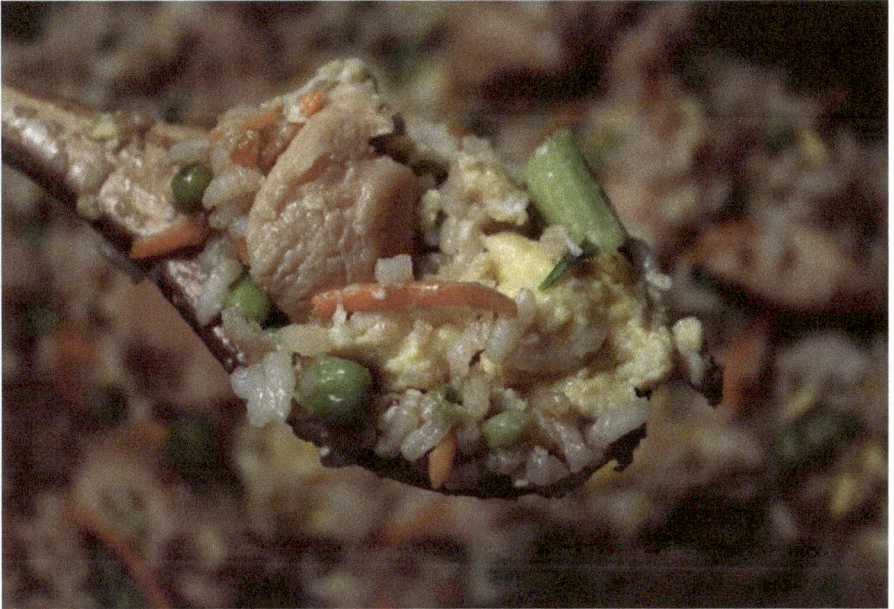

Asian-style Chicken with Vegetables

Prep Time:
35 minutes
Serve: 4

Ingredients:

- 1 lb chicken, cut in stripes
- 2 tomatoes, cubed
- 3 green peppers, cut in stripes
- 1 tbsp cumin powder
- 1 large onion
- 2 tbsp oil
- 1 tbsp mustard
- A pinch of ginger
- A pinch of fresh and chopped coriander
- Salt and black pepper

Directions:

1.Heat the oil in a deep pan.

2.Add the mustard, the onion, the ginger, the cumin and the green chili peppers.

3.Sauté the mixture for 2-3 minutes. Then, add the tomatoes, the coriander and salt and keep stirring.

4.Preheat the Air Fryer to 380 F. Coat the chicken with oil, salt and pepper and cook it for 25 minutes.

5.Remove from the Air Fryer and pour the sauce over and around.

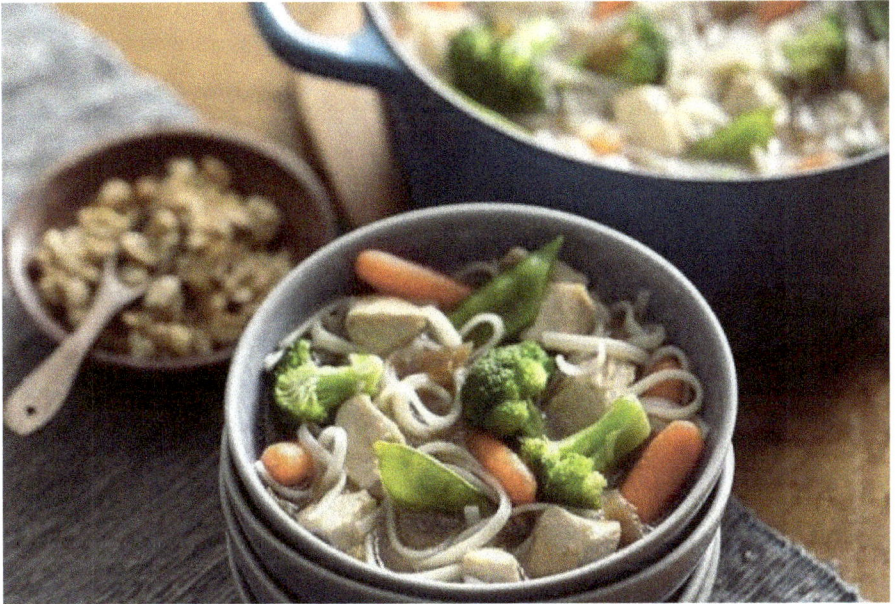

Southwest-Style Buttermilk Chicken Thighs

Prep Time:
4 hrs 40 minutes
Serve: 6

Ingredients:

- 1 ½ lb chicken thighs
- 1 tbsp cayenne pepper
- 3 tbsp salt divided
- 2 cups flour
- 2 tbsp black pepper
- 1 tbsp paprika
- 1 tbsp baking powder
- 2 cups buttermilk

Directions:

1.Rinse and pat dry the chicken thighs. Place the chicken thighs in a bowl.

2.Add cayenne pepper, 2 tbsp of salt, black pepper and buttermilk, and stir to coat well. Refrigerate for 4 hours. Preheat the air fryer to 350 F.

3.In another bowl, mix the flour, paprika, 1 tbsp of salt, and baking powder.

4.Dredge half of the chicken thighs, one at a time, in the flour, and then place on a lined dish.

5.Cook for 10 minutes, flip over and cook for 8 more minutes. Repeat with the other batch.

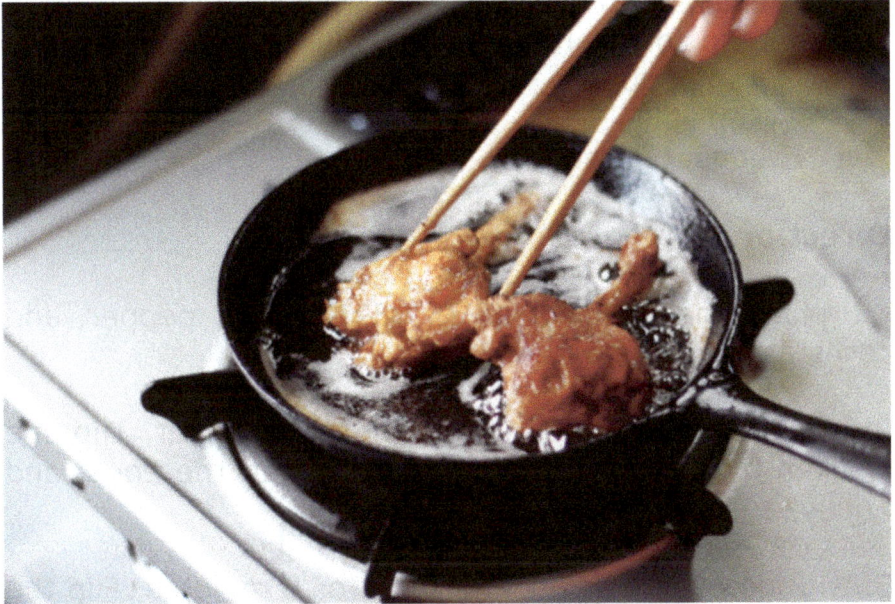

Coconut Crunch Chicken Strips

Prep Time:
22 minutes
Serve: 4

Ingredients:

- 3 ½ cups coconut flakes
- 4 chicken breasts cut into strips
- ½ cup cornstarch
- ¼ tsp pepper
- ¼ tsp salt
- 3 eggs, beaten

Directions:

1.Preheat the Air fryer to 350 F. Mix salt, pepper, and cornstarch in a small bowl.

2.Line a baking sheet with parchment paper. Dip the chicken first in the cornstarch, then into the eggs, and finally, coat with coconut flakes.

3.Arrange on the sheet and cook for 8 minutes. Flip the chicken over, and cook for 8 more minutes, until crispy.

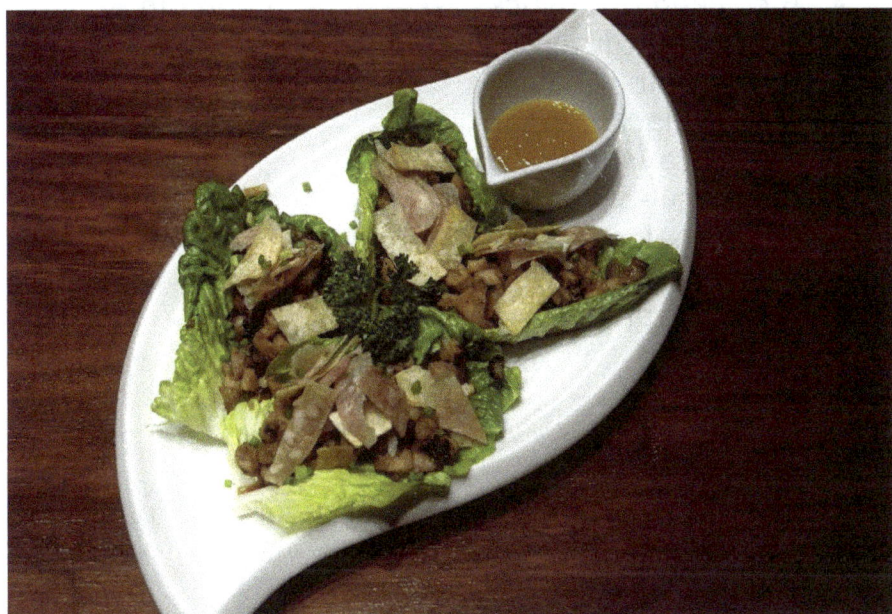

American-Style Buttermilk Fried Chicken

Prep Time:
30 minutes
Serve: 4

Ingredients:

- 6 chicken drumsticks, skin on and bone in
- 2 cups buttermilk
- 2 tbsp salt
- 2 tbsp black pepper
- 1 tbsp cayenne pepper
- 2 cups all-purpose flour
- 1 tbsp baking powder
- 1 tbsp garlic powder
- 1 tbsp paprika
- 1 tbsp salt

Directions:

1.Rinse chicken thoroughly underwater and pat them dry; remove any fat residue.

2.In a large bowl, mix paprika, black pepper and chicken. Toss well to coat the chicken evenly.

3.Pour buttermilk over chicken and toss to coat.

4.Let the chicken chill overnight. Preheat your Air Fryer to 400 F. In another bowl, mix flour, paprika, pepper and salt. Roll the chicken in the seasoned flour.

5.Place the chicken in the cooking basket in a single layer and cook for 10 minutes. Repeat the same steps for the other pieces.

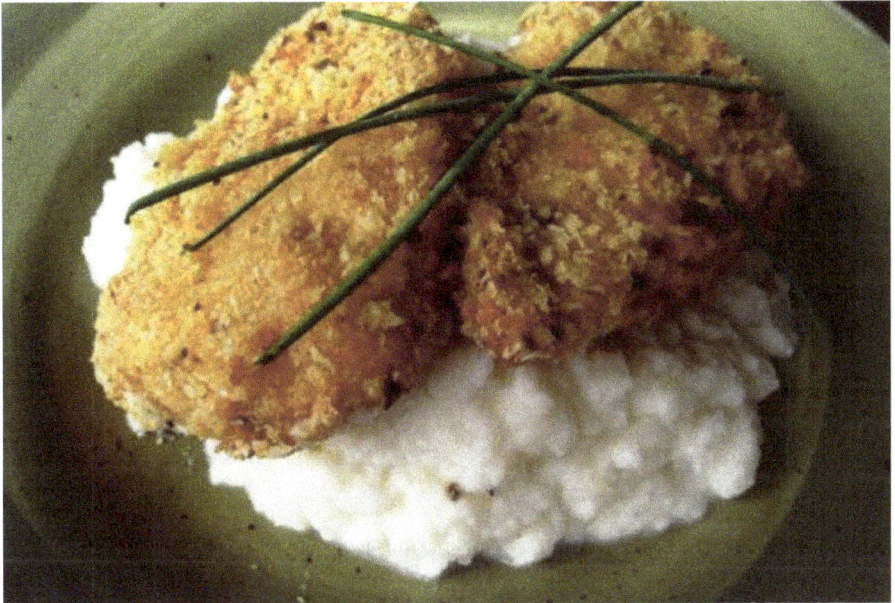

Chicken With Parmesan and Sage

Prep Time:
12 minutes
Serve: 4

Ingredients:

- 4 chicken breasts, skinless and boneless
- 3 oz breadcrumbs
- 2 tbsp grated Parmesan cheese
- 2 oz flour
- 2 eggs, beaten
- 1 tbsp fresh, chopped sage

Directions:

1.Preheat the air fryer to 370 F. Place some plastic wrap underneath and on top of the chicken breasts.

2.Using a rolling pin, beat the meat until it becomes really thin. In a bowl, combine the Parmesan cheese, sage and breadcrumbs.

3.Dip the chicken in the egg first, and then in the sage mixture.

4.Spray with cooking oil and arrange the meat in the air fryer. Cook for 7 minutes.

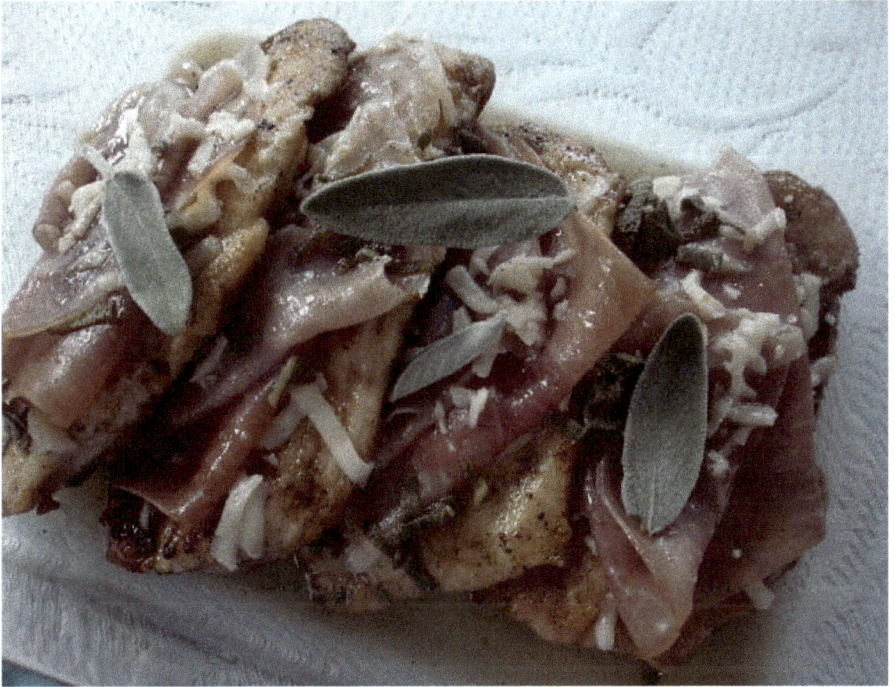

www.ingramcontent.com/pod-product-compliance
Lightning Source LLC
Chambersburg PA
CBHW061901020426
42338CB00003B/466